BLOOD POLICY

A conference sponsored by the
American Enterprise Institute for Public Policy Research

BLOOD POLICY:
ISSUES AND ALTERNATIVES

Edited by David B. Johnson

American Enterprise Institute for Public Policy Research
Washington, D.C.

Library of Congress Cataloging in Publication Data

Conference on Blood Policy, Washington, D.C., 1976.
  Blood policy.

  Papers presented at a conference sponsored by the
American Enterprise Institute.
    1. Blood banks—United States—Congresses.
I. Johnson, David B. II. American Enterprise Insti-
tute for Public Policy Research. III. Title.
RM172.C64   1976   362.1   77-10995
ISBN 0-8447-2105-0
ISBN 0-8447-2104-2 (cloth bound)

Printed in the United States of America

MAJOR CONTRIBUTORS

Ronald H. Coase
Professor of Economics, University of Chicago

John J. Corson
President, American Blood Commission

A. J. Culyer
Assistant Director
Institute of Social and Economic Research
University of York

Alvin W. Drake
Professor of Systems Science and Engineering
Massachusetts Institute of Technology

David J. Gocke, M.D.
Professor of Medicine, Rutgers Medical School

Clark C. Havighurst
Professor of Law, School of Law
Duke University

Timm M. Hurst
Executive Vice President, Blood Services

David B. Johnson
Professor of Economics
Louisiana State University

Aaron Kellner, M.D.
Director, The New York Blood Center

Louanne Kennedy
Assistant Professor of Sociology
New York University

Arthur N. Levine
Associate Chief Counsel for Biologics
Food and Drug Administration

Harry M. Meyer, Jr., M.D.
Director, Bureau of Biologics
Food and Drug Administration

Ian Mitchell, M.D.
Special Assistant to the Assistant Secretary
Department of Health, Education, and Welfare

Herbert F. Polesky, M.D.
Director, The Minneapolis War Memorial Blood Bank

Mike Reddin
Lecturer in Social Administration
The London School of Economics and Political Science

Simon Rottenberg
Professor of Economics
University of Massachusetts

Gordon Tullock
Professor of Economics
Virginia Polytechnic Institute

Edward L. Wallace
Chairman, Department of Management Systems
State University of New York, Buffalo

Irwin J. Wargon
Lecturer in Economics
California State University, Fullerton

CONTENTS

PART THREE

Current Practices and Suggested Reforms

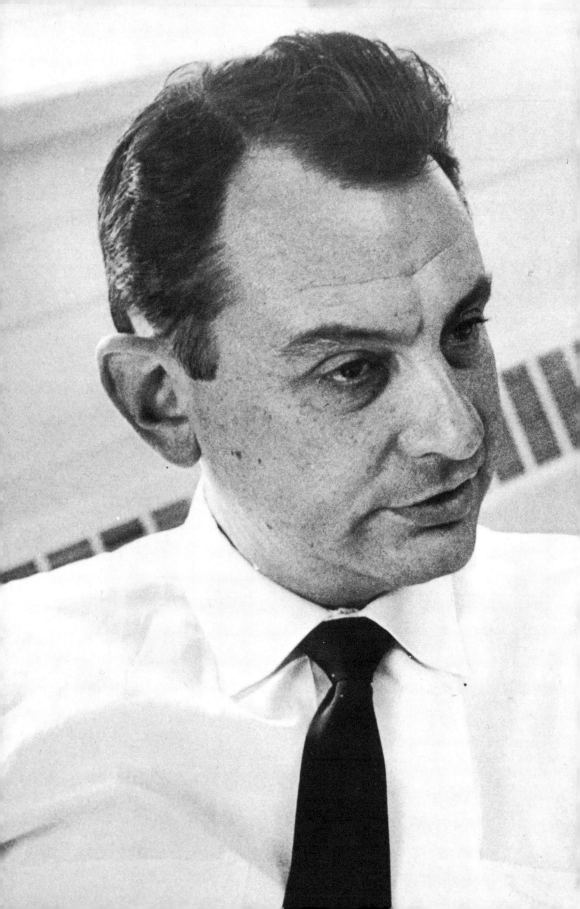

DEDICATION TO PROFESSOR REUBEN KESSEL

Ronald H. Coase

It is an honor for me to be asked to dedicate this important conference on blood policy to Reuben Kessel. Reuben Kessel was to have taken part in this conference, but was prevented from doing so by his untimely death, a grievous loss to all his friends and a heavy blow to the world of scholarship.

Reuben Kessel was a natural-born economist. He did not start with theory, as is so common today, but rather with a problem. And his analysis was always custom-built to increase our understanding of the particular problem with which he was dealing.

He had an intense and longstanding interest in health economics, and his contributions to this subject earned him a respected position in this branch of economics. He enhanced his reputation with what was unfortunately to prove to be his last major paper, that on transfused blood and serum hepatitis.

As in all Reuben Kessel's work, his argument is not hedged around with qualifications. Like a chess master, he aimed to win, but was quite willing to make himself vulnerable to do so.

It is a great loss to those of us attending this conference that Reuben Kessel could not take part in our proceedings. He would have been an active participant and his contributions forceful and to the point. However, a scholar of Reuben Kessel's distinction lives on in his works. And whether one agrees or disagrees with his arguments, it is a mark of his distinction that his views cannot be ignored.

We cannot ask that a scholar present us with the whole truth. That is something which eludes us all. The most we can expect is that we know more after studying his work than we knew before.

Alfred Marshall once wrote of those whose ideas, once created, can never die; but are an existing yeast ceaselessly working in the cosmos. Reuben Kessel was one of those rare scholars who belong in this category. Mrs. Shirley Kessel is with us today and though nothing we can say can touch her sense of deep personal loss, it may make it more bearable for her to know that the flame Reuben Kessel lit will not be extinguished.

INTRODUCTION:
THE BLOOD MARKET

David B. Johnson

Blood is a juice of the rarest quality.
Goethe, *Faust*

The brain may devise laws for the blood,
but a hot temper leaps o'er a cold decree.
Shakespeare, *The Merchant of Venice*

Although the average citizen probably gives much less thought to the supply of blood than he does to the supply of table salt, the process of procuring and distributing blood involves a plethora of social policy issues and administrative problems. It also offers, to anyone who immerses himself in the subject, more than a modicum of intellectual excitement. Historically, the blood market has been an almost exclusive province of medical doctors and professional blood bankers, but within the past five years donor groups, consumers, journalists, and government regulators have begun taking an interest—and, more important, an active role—in the blood market.

Blood is a unique resource in the human body, the "vehicle" that carries oxygen, nutrients, and chemicals to all parts of the body and carries away waste products. Human blood cannot be replaced by chemical substitutes or by the blood of other animals; thus, all whole-blood transfusion and the increasingly large number of drugs derived from the components of blood are dependent upon the commercial or volunteer donor. Blood is composed of several components or fractions which have different medical uses in the treatment of patients. These components include red and white cells, salt, water, sugars, fats, and proteins. Whole blood is generally given to patients who have suffered massive blood losses or who are undergoing such specialized operations as open-heart surgery. In an increasing number of cases, doctors are utilizing only the red blood cells instead of whole blood. The noncellular component of blood, a yellow liquid called plasma, is medically nearly as important as the cellular components. It contains fibrogen and other coagulation factors; albumin, which tends to draw fluid into the blood, a critical factor in maintaining the volume of circulating blood; and globulins, some of which are antibodies. These components are used to produce numerous drug derivatives, which have a multitude of applications. Plasma is

1

obtained from donors through a process called *plasmapheresis* which separates the liquid portion of the blood from the cellular portion and then returns the cellular portion to the donor.

There are numerous and important distinctions between the segments of the blood market dealing with whole blood and red cells on the one hand and plasma on the other. First, an individual can give two units of plasma as often as twice a week, whereas he can give whole blood only five times a year. Second, whole blood and red cells will be subject to the Food and Drug Administration's proposed labeling regulations, whereas plasma will not be. Third, the whole-blood red-cell segment of the blood market will be subject to the new National Blood Policy's goal of an all-volunteer (whole) blood supply, whereas the plasma segment will not be. Fourth, the institutional organization of the blood market is sharply segmented by the whole-blood plasma distinction. Virtually all of the 6 million pints of plasma obtained annually in the United States are collected through the plasmapheresis process either by commercial plasma centers, which then sell to pharmaceutical firms or directly by the drug firms, which use plasma to manufacture drug derivatives. Other sources of plasma are outdated whole blood and the plasma residual that is a byproduct of red-cell-component therapy. Although numerous questions are being raised about the plasma segment of the blood market and the role of the pharmaceutical industry in it, this volume is concerned primarily with the other segment of the blood market, that is, the segment concerned with whole blood and red blood cells. The remainder of this paper presents an overview of the whole-blood red-cell submarket.

Nearly 11 million pints of whole blood were drawn from donors in the United States during 1976. Because of its normal twenty-one-day shelf life and the blood banks' desire to maintain a "margin of safety" in their blood inventories, only about 75 to 80 percent of the blood drawn from donors is actually transfused into patients. The whole-blood red-cell segment of the blood market consists of a complex series of interrelated national and local profit and nonprofit institutions. Approximately 40 percent of the blood supply is drawn by the American Red Cross (ARC), 40 percent by independent members of the American Association of Blood Banks (AABB), 10 percent by members of the Council of Community Blood Banks (CCBB), and approximately 10 percent by commercial blood banks. Until fairly recently, the fifty-eight Red Cross blood centers were members of AABB's clearinghouse system which processes donor credits for donors replacing blood used for friends or relatives and for donors who are members of blood assurance or insurance systems. The Red Cross withdrew from the clearinghouse in October 1976.

Virtually all blood banks, including the ARC, charge hospitals a fee for processing blood, which is intended to cover the costs of personnel, equipment, and supplies involved in the collection, laboratory testing, storage, and distribution of blood. Most members of AABB generally add a "replacement" or "recruitment" fee (generally in the range of twenty to forty dollars) that is passed on to the patient unless he, his friends, or his family "replace" the blood transfused. The official philosophy of the Red Cross and a few other community blood banks is that the blood supply is a "community" responsibility and that a patient should receive blood without having to pay a replacement fee, regardless whether he predeposited or whether his friends or family donate blood. Blood bankers have very strong and divisive views about the equity and efficiency of "individual" versus "community" responsibility.

Controversies and Legal Responses

The (whole) blood market has always had its share of problems and controversies, but in recent years these seem to have been increasing in importance and number. A considerable number of these problems and controversies are related to two factors: one is the difference between the incidence of post-transfusion hepatitis (PTH) related to the use of so-called paid or commercial blood and that related to the use of volunteer blood; and the other is the existence of competing philosophies pertaining to the responsibility for the provision of blood.

During the past thirty years, but especially within the last decade, evidence has strongly suggested that, on the average, the incidence of post-transfusion hepatitis is considerably higher in patients who have received transfusions of commercial blood than in those who have received transfusions of volunteer blood. Although third-generation tests utilizing the hepatitis B antigen and sensitive screening procedures do exist for testing donor hepatitis infectivity, the tests screen out only about 50 to 60 percent of type B hepatitis carriers. More recent medical research has discovered the existence of a non-A, non-B post-transfusion hepatitis for which there are no suitable testing procedures.

Given the inability of the tests to detect 100 percent of the hepatitis carriers, the discovery of the relationship between commercial blood and the incidence of PTH significantly contributed to the establishment of state blood-labeling laws, the National Blood Policy, and the proposed blood-labeling regulations of the Food and Drug Administration. The first state to pass a labeling law was Illinois, with the enactment of its Blood Labeling Act on October 1, 1972. This law requires that blood be labeled either volunteer or purchased and that, when purchased blood is used, the physician make a written notation on the patient's chart explaining the necessity of using it. In 1976, California and Georgia passed similar blood-labeling acts.

At the national level, the epidemiological studies pertaining to hepatitis incidence were only one of the developments that prompted HEW to investigate the U.S. blood market in the early 1970s. Another was the influence of *The Gift Relationship*, a book published in 1970 by Richard Titmuss, a social philosopher working at the London School of Economics. Titmuss argued that the British altruistic

3

blood system had social and medical advantages over the U.S. commercial system. Yet another spur was the existence of nearly forty pieces of pending blood-market legislation in Congress. In December 1971, HEW Secretary Richardson asked Dr. Ian Mitchell, special assistant secretary of health, to assemble a staff to develop a national blood policy. Based on the work of this committee and subsequent government conferences, the National Blood Policy, which espoused the goal of creating an all-volunteer blood system, was announced in the *Federal Register* of July 10, 1973. In September 1973, the Department of Health, Education, and Welfare requested the aid of the blood-banking community in implementing the operational aspects of the National Blood Policy. The blood-banking sector responded by proposing the creation of the American Blood Commission. HEW approved the creation of the American Blood Commission (ABC) in September 1974.

ABC comprises organizations representing blood banks, hospitals, users, donors, and the medical profession as well as professional individuals. In 1975 the American Blood Resource Association (ABRA), an association of commercial blood banks, filed a suit against HEW and ABC in an effort to abolish the ABC. ABRA's major legal argument was that HEW did not possess the statutory authority to create the American Blood Commission. The suit was dismissed in the district court but it is now being appealed.

A second prong of federal policy pertaining to the whole-blood market came from the Food and Drug Administration in November 1975, when it published in the *Federal Register* the *Proposed Rules and Regulations on Whole Blood and Red Blood Cells: Label Statement to Distinguish Volunteer from Paid Blood Donors*. Like the Illinois labeling law, the FDA proposal required that all whole blood or red cells be labeled "volunteer" or "paid" and that labels on paid blood state that it carried a higher risk of hepatitis. The FDA argued that such labeling would reduce the incidence of post-transfusion hepatitis and would reinforce the National Blood Policy's goal of an all-volunteer blood supply. The FDA's proposed regulations received considerable criticism for not appropriately defining *volunteer* and *paid* and for requiring all paid blood to carry the health warning. Many blood banks that utilize paid blood, such as the Mayo Clinic in Minnesota, argued that their commercial blood was of a higher quality than volunteer blood. The most significant reaction, however, came from the Council on Wage and Price Stability (COWPS), a small but very active federal agency. The council not only commented on the FDA's labeling regulations but also argued that an all-volunteer blood program would be inflationary. Many of the council's analytical and empirical arguments were based on the arguments formulated by the late Professor Reuben Kessel in his article "Transfused Blood, Serum Hepatitis, and the Coase Theorem," which, because of its importance to the debate, is reprinted in this volume as Appendix B. The COWPS statement, which was the first widely publicized attack on the concept of an all-volunteer blood program, received strong

4

criticism from the ABC, the FDA, HEW, and some sectors of the nonprofit blood-banking industry.

One of the major purposes of this conference was to enable blood bankers, doctors, lawyers, economists, and government officials to exchange views on the recent controversies arising within the blood market. Even a cursory reading of the conference papers and comments contained in this volume will suggest that views differ both among and within the professions. Many of the participants were unfamiliar with the analyses and arguments of professionals outside of their own fields and, although the exchange of ideas among rational men did not produce a Rousseauistic consensus, it may have fissured the walls surrounding the separate professional and ideological enclaves.

Part One of this volume explores the blood market from the viewpoint of medicine, law, and economics. Part Two presents an address by Dr. Harry Meyer, Jr., who, as director of the Bureau of Biologics, is actively engaged in the federal regulation of blood banking. Part Three presents the results of research by two academicians and a plea for a change in social policy on blood by the director of one of this country's most progressive blood centers.

I would like to extend my appreciation to the American Enterprise Institute for sponsoring this conference and publishing this volume and to Robert Helms, director of AEI's Center for Health Policy Research, Linda Eiben, and Faith Breen of AEI for their assistance in planning and organizing the conference as well as to Linda Teekel of Louisiana State University for her dedicated secretarial and typing assistance in organizing the conference and in editing this volume.

PART ONE

MEDICAL, LEGAL, AND ECONOMIC ASPECTS OF BLOOD

CHAIRMAN'S COMMENTS

Ronald H. Coase

Part One of the American Enterprise Institute's Conference on Blood Policy proved to be lively and informative. The discussion concentrated on three main issues: (1) Should there be either a wholly or partially commercial market for blood? (2) What should be the liability of the various parties involved in the collection and distribution of blood? (3) What is the importance of the transmission of serum hepatitis in the process of blood transfusion and what are its implications for policy?

The discussion of these questions is difficult because, in dealing with each of them, there are medical, economic, and legal issues to be resolved. This must have created a problem for the participants, whose expertise was inevitably mainly in one field, but it was one which in fact they surmounted with ease.

The discussion was, however, complicated by another factor. For many participants the answer they would give to the first and second of the basic questions under consideration depended on the answers that were given to the other questions. To decide what the effects would be of allowing a market in blood, and therefore whether there should be such a market, could well depend on what the position was assumed to be regarding the liability of the parties for the harm or injury resulting from a blood transfusion and may also depend on the extent to which the risk of transmitting serum hepatitis along with the blood varied among various groups in the population. Of course, it can be argued, and was in this session by Mike Reddin, that there should not be a market for blood, whatever the position was regarding liability or the incidence of serum hepatitis; but this was not, I would judge, the view of most participants. Similarly, it is possible to discuss the problem of liability whether or not there is a market in blood or whatever the position may be regarding serum hepatitis, but one's conclusion about what the law ought to be is likely to be influenced by whether there is a market or by the seriousness of the risk of contracting serum hepatitis. Such interrelationships between the questions under discussion undoubtedly made the task of exposition more difficult for all participants.

As has been said earlier, the major policy questions can be discussed without regard to the character of the serum hepatitis problem, but it is hardly possible to come to a conclusion about them without taking it into account. It was therefore

9

appropriate that the first paper of the session was a status report on serum hepatitis by Dr. David J. Gocke. Professor A. J. Culyer informed the conference of the state of the debate over blood policy among social scientists, and Professor Havighurst explained the complexities of the law and made a critical appraisal of the current legal position. Participants in the conference were thus enabled to examine blood policy with all the relevant background information before them. If the ensuing discussion cannot be said to have resolved the issues, there can be no doubt that the main papers and the contributions of the discussants went a long way towards clarifying what the choices are that we have to make and what the factors are on which these choices should depend.

POST-TRANSFUSION HEPATITIS: A STATUS REPORT

David J. Gocke

Since the basic problems of cross-matching and preserving blood were overcome, post-transfusion hepatitis (PTH) has stood out as the major complication of blood transfusion by whatever measure one chooses—mortality, morbidity, or economic impact on the individual and society. The problem has increased in recent years as a result of the increased use of blood in connection with advanced and complicated surgical techniques and other forms of therapy which tend to keep sicker people alive for longer periods of time. In addition, the widespread social problem of drug abuse has had an impact on the problem by increasing the reservoir of hepatitis in the blood-donor population.

It has now been approximately ten years since Blumberg and his colleagues first described Australia antigen, now referred to as the hepatitis B surface antigen, or HB_sAg.[1] Two or three years were required to demonstrate convincingly a relationship between this antigen and serum hepatitis or post-transfusion hepatitis. Originally it was anticipated that this discovery would eventually lead to universal exclusion of blood donors with this hepatitis factor and result in total solution of the problem of PTH. But this initial hope has not been borne out. The purpose of this presentation is to give a status report on PTH. The points to be considered are:

(1) The current incidence of PTH. Has the screening of blood for the HB_sAg really reduced the incidence of this disease?

(2) The current understanding of the etiologic agents responsible for this disease. What is now known or thought about type B, non-type B, and possible type C hepatitis viruses?

(3) The status of current test methodologies.

(4) The status of "commercial" versus "volunteer" blood.

(5) An update on the present status of potential vaccines for hepatitis.

---

[1] Baruch S. Blumberg, B. J. S. Grestley, D. A. Hungerford et al., "A Serum Antigen (Australia Antigen) on Down's Syndrome, Leukemia, and Hepatitis," *Annals of Internal Medicine*, vol. 66 (December 1967), pp. 924-31.

Causative Agents

Table 1 supplies some basic orientation material for those not intimately familiar with the field. By way of general introduction, we have thought in terms of two classical types of hepatitis—type A and type B. Type A, previously called infectious hepatitis, is usually transmitted by the fecal-to-oral route and is responsible for most episodes of hepatitis associated with ingestion of contaminated water or seafood. In contrast, type B, or "serum hepatitis," has classically been thought to be transmitted only by inoculation or by blood transfusion and until recently was thought to be the primary cause of post-transfusion hepatitis.

Figure 1 is an electron micrograph of the hepatitis B virus. The hepatitis B

Table 1
CHARACTERISTICS OF VIRAL HEPATITIS TYPES A AND B

Characteristic	Type A	Type B
Synonyms	Infectious hepatitis, short-incubation hepatitis	Serum hepatitis, long-incubation hepatitis
Transmission		
Usual	Fecal-oral	Parenteral
Alternative	Parenteral?	Frequently nonparenteral (salivary? venereal?)
Incubation period	2 to 6 weeks	6 weeks to 6 months
Severity	Usually mild, often anicteric	Often severe, usually icteric, long period of morbidity
Distribution	Point source outbreaks, random cases	Prevalent in young adults and urban populations
Chronic disease	?	Accounts for about 30% of cases of chronic hepatitis
Carrier state	?	20-30% of cases of infection result in carrier state
Gamma globulin prophylaxis	Ordinary pooled globulin highly effective	Specific hepatitis B immune globulin effective in some selected settings
Serologic markers	HA Ag, anti-HA	HB_sAg, anti-HB_s HB_cAg, anti-HB_c

Note: HB_sAg, hepatitis B surface antigen; anti-HB_s, antibody to surface antigen; HB_cAg, hepatitis B core antigen; anti-HB_c, antibody to core antigen; HA Ag, hepatitis A antigen; anti-HA, antibody to hepatitis A antigen.
Source: Modified from David J. Gocke, "Viral Hepatitis," *Postgraduate Medicine*, vol. 58, no. 3 (September 1975), pp. 137-42.

Figure 1

ELECTRON MICROGRAPH OF HEPATITIS A VIRUS

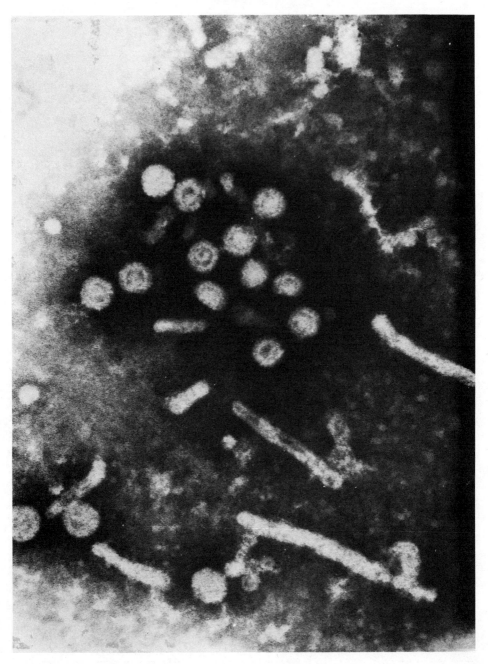

Figure 2
ELECTRON MICROGRAPH OF HEPATITIS B VIRUS

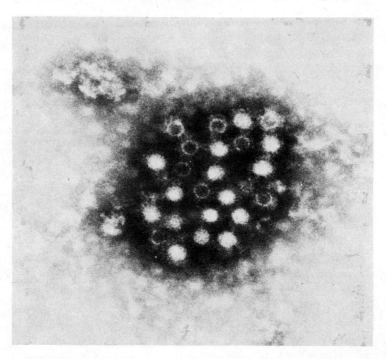

surface antigen has been shown to be the external lipoprotein coat of this virus. It is this material that is detected in the serum of the patient with hepatitis or the infectious donor and is used as a marker of the presence of the virus. Figure 2 is an electron micrograph of type A hepatitis virus. This is a totally different agent for which there is no widely available serologic test at the present time. Although the presence of type A antigen can be demonstrated in the research laboratory, the technology for its detection is not yet available at a practical level.

It became apparent early in our studies of the relation of HB_sAg to post-transfusion hepatitis that the presence of this antigen was a reliable indicator of the infectivity of the donor blood. Table 2 summarizes data collected by my laboratory in New York City between 1968 and 1971.[2] Approximately 75 percent of recipients of blood from donors who were positive for the antigen exhibited evidence of hepatitis B infection. This kind of data was corroborated by several other laboratories at the time and established the point that HB_sAg was a reliable marker of infectivity and led to the universal screening of donors for the presence

[2] David J. Gocke, "A Prospective Study of Post-Transfusion Hepatitis: The Role of Australia Antigen," *Journal of the American Medical Association*, vol. 219 (1972), pp. 1165-70.

Table 2

POST-TRANSFUSION HEPATITIS IN RECIPIENTS OF HB_sAg POSITIVE OR NEGATIVE BLOOD, 1968-1971

Donor Status	No. of Recipients	Result of Transfusion				
		Ag-Positive Hepatitis	Ag-Negative Hepatitis	HB_sAg Only	Anti-HB_sAg	Well
Positive	84	21	14	9	19	21
Negative	82	1	15	0	1	65

Source: David J. Gocke, "A Prospective Study of Post-Transfusion Hepatitis: The Role of Australia Antigen," *Journal of the American Medical Association*, vol. 219 (1972), pp. 1165-70.

of this antigen.[3] However, note that in the control group—that is, recipients of HB_sAg-negative blood—a significant number also developed hepatitis. The rate was markedly lower than among the recipients of positive blood; nevertheless fifteen out of eighty-two developed hepatitis that was HB_sAg negative in the acute phase. This raised the question whether some cases of PTH were caused by other viral agents (that is, non-type B) or whether small amounts of HB_sAg had escaped detection in some units of apparently negative donor blood. In order to answer this question, apparently negative donor units that had been transfused into individuals who subsequently developed hepatitis were retrieved from storage. When these donors were retested by the most sensitive radioimmunoassay, it was discovered that only 28 percent (five out of eighteen cases) could be attributed to missed weakly positive donor units (see Table 3).[4] But there remained a number of type B PTH cases (72 percent) that could not have been recognized in spite of the application of the most sensitive test methods available. Furthermore, there were ten individuals who developed HB_sAg-negative hepatitis following a blood transfusion in which hepatitis B virus could not be implicated (see Table 3), again suggesting the existence of so-called non-type B PTH. Similar data have come from a number of laboratories.[5]

---

[3] K. Ohochi, S. Murakami, K. Ninomiya et al., "Australia Antigen, Transfusion and Hepatitis," *Vox Sanguinis*, vol. 18 (September/October 1970), pp. 289-300; Paul V. Holland, Harvey J. Alter, Robert H. Purcell et al., "The Infectivity of Blood Containing the Australia Antigen," in *Australia Antigen*, J. E. Prier and H. Friedman, eds. (Baltimore: University Park Press, 1973), pp. 191-203; David J. Gocke, Harry B. Grunberg, Neal B. Kavey, "Correlation of Australia Antigen with Post-Transfusion Hepatitis," *Journal of the American Medical Association*, vol. 212 (September/October 1970), pp. 877-79.

[4] David J. Gocke and Zarah F. Kachani, "Solid-Phase Radioimmunoassay for Hepatitis B Antigen," *Journal of the American Medical Association*, vol. 224 (June 1973), p. 1426.

[5] Harvey J. Alter, Paul V. Holland, Robert H. Purcell et al., "Post-Transfusion Hepatitis after Exclusion of the Commercial and Hepatitis B Antigen Positive Donor," *Annals of Internal Medicine*, vol. 77 (November 1972), pp. 691-99; Alfred M. Prince, Betsy Brotman, George F. Grady et al., "Long-Incubation Post-Transfusion Hepatitis without Serologic Evidence of Exposure to Hepatitis B Virus," *Lancet*, vol. 2 (1974), pp. 241-46.

Table 3

DETECTION OF HB$_s$Ag BY RADIOIMMUNOASSAY IN APPARENTLY NEGATIVE DONORS IMPLICATED IN POST-TRANSFUSION HEPATITIS

Result of Transfusion	No. of Cases	No. of Cases Associated with an RIA-Positive Donor
HB$_s$AG-positive hepatitis	18	5
HB$_s$Ag-negative hepatitis	10	0
No hepatitis	26	0

Source: David J. Gocke and Zarah F. Kachani, "Solid-Phase Radioimmunoassay for Hepatitis B Antigen," *Journal of the American Medical Association*, vol. 224 (June 1973), p. 1426.

The Impact of Screening for the Hepatitis B Antigen. In light of the above, let us consider what has happened to the incidence of post-transfusion hepatitis since the discovery of the hepatitis B antigen and the introduction of sensitive screening tests into the blood bank. The study by Seeff and his colleagues from a collaborative Veterans Administration study provides one of the clearest opportunities to compare the incidence of PTH within the same setting between the years 1969 and 1974.[6] Since 1973, when the more sensitive third-generation tests for hepatitis B antigen were introduced, the VA experience shows a modest gradual decline in the overall incidence of PTH.

Table 4 is a composite extracted from data reported by several different groups of investigators concerning the problem of post-transfusion hepatitis. The incidence of hepatitis is given for two periods—"then" and "now." "Then" is the period before intensive screening for hepatitis B antigen by any methodology was introduced, and generally these data come from the period before 1969. In contrast, the "now" period is the time since the widespread institution of sensitive radioimmunoassay methods. Notice that "now" the reported incidence of hepatitis ranges between the 5 percent seen by Aach and his collaborators in St. Louis to as high as 28 percent reported by Goldfield and his colleagues in New Jersey. These are figures for the overall incidence of all types of post-transfusion hepatitis. Cases which can be attributed to the type B virus still occur, but they represent a small fraction of the overall problem. As shown in Table 4, type B hepatitis was seen in only 0 to 2.6 percent of recipients, and at worst accounts for only about 30 percent of *all* cases of PTH (see data of Hollinger et al.).

The current experience, then, could be summarized thus: It would appear that

[6] Leonard B. Seeff, Elizabeth C. Wright, Hyman J. Zimmerman et al., "VA Cooperative Study of Post-Transfusion Hepatitis, 1969-1974: Incidence and Characteristics of Hepatitis and Reasonable Risk Factors," *American Journal of Medical Science*, vol. 270 (September/October 1975), pp. 355-62.

Table 4

POST-TRANSFUSION HEPATITIS—THEN AND NOW

| | | Incidence of Hepatitis in Transfusion Recipients (in percentages) | | | |
| | | Then[a] | | Now[b] | |
Investigators	Origin of Blood	All types	Hepa- titis B[c]	All types	Hepa- titis B[c]
Aach et al.	All volunteer	10.0	—	5.4	0
Alter et al.	Mixed to all volunteer	51.0	—	11.0	0.9
Goldfield et al.	Volunteer	—	—	8.5	1.4
	Commercial	—	—	28.7	2.0
Hollinger et al.	Mixed	—	—	8.7	2.6
Seeff et al.	Mixed	10.4	2.3	10.5	0.7

a Before HB$_s$Ag screening was introduced—generally, before 1969.
b Since the widespread institution of RIA screening for HB$_s$Ag.
c The figures shown for hepatitis B represent the incidence of cases specifically attributable to type B infection.
Source: L. B. Seeff, E. C. Wright, H. J. Zimmerman et al., "VA Cooperative Study of Post-Transfusion Hepatitis, 1969-1974: Incidence and Characteristics of Hepatitis and Responsible Risk Factors," *American Journal of Medical Science*, vol. 270 (September/October 1975), pp. 355-62; H. J. Alter, P. V. Holland, and R. H. Purcell, "The Emerging Pattern of Post-Transfusion Hepatitis," ibid., pp. 329-34; M. Goldfield, H. C. Black, J. Bill et al., "The Consequences of Administering Blood Pretested for HB$_s$Ag by Third Generation Techniques: A Progress Report," ibid., pp. 335-42; F. B. Hollinger, G. R. Dreesman, H. Fields et al., "HB$_c$Ag, Anti-HB$_c$, and DNA Polymerase Activity in Transfused Recipients Followed Prospectively," ibid., pp. 343-48; R. D. Aach et al., Discussion of Post-Transfusion Hepatitis, National Academy of Sciences Symposium on Viral Hepatitis, March 1975.

there has been a reduction of only approximately 50 percent in the overall incidence of PTH despite the application of the most sensitive technology for HB$_s$Ag detection. PTH continues to occur in from 5 to 28 percent of recipients, with a mean of about 10 to 15 percent. Furthermore, about 10 to 15 percent of all PTH continues to be caused by the type B virus. This has led to the realization that much PTH is not due to the type B virus and again suggests the existence of other non-type B hepatitis viruses. Recent attempts to demonstrate that cases of non-type B PTH are due to type A virus have failed.[7] Hence the suggestion that some previously unrecognized viral agent or agents can produce PTH—the putative type C hepatitis virus. At present there are no techniques available for the detection of these other viruses and the evidence for their existence is circumstantial.

7 Stephen M. Feinstone, Albert Z. Kapikian, Robert H. Purcell et al., "Transfusion Associated Hepatitis Not Due to Viral Hepatitis Type A or B," *New England Journal of Medicine*, vol. 292 (February 1975), pp. 454-57.

High-Risk and Low-Risk Blood. Now a word about "volunteer" and "commercial" blood donors. Several studies have documented a lower incidence of PTH associated with the use of so-called volunteer donors as compared with the incidence associated with paid donors. The importance of this consideration is demonstrated again by the Veterans Administration study mentioned above. In one Veterans Administration hospital where there was a reduction in 1973 in the percentage of so-called paid donors from 91 percent to 4 percent, there was a coincident drop-off in the rate of PTH from 20 percent to 6 percent. However, the data currently being reported, such as that from Goldfield et al. in New Jersey (Table 5), indicate that, while volunteer blood is associated with a lower incidence of PTH as compared with commercial blood (8 percent versus 28 percent), one still sees a significant rate of PTH even when volunteer blood is used. Thus, it is incorrect to imply that blood obtained from a volunteer source os totally safe for transfusion.

Personally, I believe the times has come for those of us in the field who have referred loosely to "commercial" donors, "paid" donors, or "volunteer" donors to begin talking in more precise terms. We should carefully define certain blood donors as "high-risk" donors, and these can be recognized by certain epidemiological characteristics which tend to be associated with the transmission of hepatitis to a recipient. In Table 6 I have listed some of these factors and divided them into minor and major categories. For example, a history of drug abuse, confinement in an institution such as a prison, previous blood transfusion, and male homosexuality are factors that are associated with a prohibitively high rate of transmission of hepatitis. Any one of these characteristics ought to exclude an individual from blood donation. In addition, with a little thought and analysis of available data, it ought to be possible to derive a composite relative risk factor based on

Table 5

INCIDENCE OF HEPATITIS IN RECIPIENTS OF RADIOIMMUNOASSAY-TESTED "VOLUNTEER" AND "COMMERCIAL" BLOOD

Origin of Blood	Transfusions Administered		Recipients with Hepatitis			
	No. of recipients	Units of blood	All	(Rate)[a]	HBV infection	(Rate)[a]
"Volunteer"	364	1,066	31	(8.5)	5	(1.37)
"Commercial"	101	233	29	(28.7)	2	(1.98)

[a] Rate per 100 recipients.
Source: M. Goldfield, H. C. Black, J. Bill et al., "The Consequences of Administering Blood Pretested for HB$_s$Ag by Third Generation Techniques," pp. 335-42.

Table 6

HEPATITIS RISK FACTORS OF BLOOD DONORS

Minor	Major
Age	Drug abuse
Sex	Previous blood transfusion
Race	Institutional confinement
Address	Male homosexuality
Occupation	
History of hepatitis	

Source: Author.

the minor characteristics shown in Table 6. This would seem to be a more rational and justifiable approach than excluding or accepting a donor on the basis of whether money changes hands.

Vaccines. Finally, a word about the present status of hepatitis vaccines. First of all, time does not permit me to present the data currently available that strongly suggest that hepatitis B immune globulin (HBIG) is protective against type B hepatitis. These studies were carried out in a variety of populations, such as patients receiving treatment in dialysis units, medical personnel experiencing accidental needle-sticks, and spouses of individuals with type B hepatitis, but do *not* come from blood-transfusion studies.[8] It is important to note in this symposium that even if there is acceptable evidence that HBIG is effective in preventing type B hepatitis in some settings, it has not yet been established that it is effective in the blood-transfusion setting. Attempts to develop subunit vaccines for active immunization to type B hepatitis virus are also underway. Several years will be required before this work can be completed. Again it should be pointed out in regard to the PTH problem that it is unlikely that any kind of active vaccine would ever satisfy the need to immunize an individual who requires transfusion on an emergency basis. At present, there is no vaccine on the horizon for type A virus, and, of course, the presumptive type C and other possible hepatitis viruses are far from being considered in this regard.

---

[8] George F. Grady and V. A. Lee, "Hepatitis B Immune Globulin: Prevention of Hepatitis from Accidental Exposures among Medical Personnel: A Preliminary Report of a Cooperative Multiantu Trial," *New England Journal of Medicine*, vol. 293 (November 1975), pp. 1067-70; Alfred M. Prince, Wolfe Szmuness, M. K. Mann et al., "Hepatitis B 'Immune' Globulin: Effectiveness in Prevention of Dialysis-Associated Hepatitis," ibid., pp. 1063-67; Allan G. Redekee, James W. Mosley, David J. Gocke et al., "Hepatitis B Immune Globulin as a Prophylactic Measure for Spouses Exposed to Acute Type B Hepatitis," ibid., pp. 1055-59; Leonard B. Seeff, Hyman J. Zimmerman, Elizabeth C. Wright et al., "Efficacy of Hepatitis B Immune Globulin after Accidental Exposure. Preliminary Report of the Veterans Administration Cooperative Study," *Lancet*, vol. 2 (November 1975), pp. 939-41.

LEGAL RESPONSES TO THE PROBLEM OF POOR-QUALITY BLOOD

Clark C. Havighurst

Four years ago I spoke at an AEI conference on the subject of health planning, considering the then relatively new phenomenon of certificate-of-need laws, which extend the public utility notion to hospitals and other health facilities. The paper I delivered ended on one of the themes which I am called upon to consider today. In that paper, I discussed the constructive role markets and competition, particularly between health maintenance organizations and the fee-for-service sector, might play in guiding the health-care delivery system toward better control of health-care costs, and I closed this otherwise mildly hopeful talk by noting "the obstacle of antimarket attitudes." I referred specifically to Professor Titmuss's attempt in his book *The Gift Relationship*[1] to attribute the poor U.S. record on post-transfusion hepatitis to an excess of "commercialism" and to extrapolate from this observation broader conclusions about the shortcomings of free markets. My remarks were as follows:

> Not only do Professor Titmuss's veiled efforts to generalize from this unique market fail, but the obvious and regrettable market failures he finds so significant [that is, the hepatitis problem] appear readily correctable without rejecting the market as the primary organizing influence. For example, a legal rule imposing strict liability for hepatitis reactions on blood banks and on hospitals would have generated closer attention not only to blood collection methods and donor selection but also to the development of blood testing techniques and to alternatives to the use of blood in therapy. Such a legal rule, which is readily derivable from recent market-oriented scholarship in the field of torts, was adopted by a number of courts but subsequently rejected by numerous legislatures to whom the hospitals quickly appealed. Nevertheless, adoption of this legal solution of creating reasonably balanced market incentives for providers to find the least-cost solution to the problem might so change the conditions studied by Professor Titmuss that his conclusions would have to be, if not reversed, at least retracted.[2]

---

[1] Richard M. Titmuss, *The Gift Relationship: From Human Blood to Social Policy* (New York: Pantheon Books, 1971).

[2] Clark C. Havighurst, "Speculations on the Market's Future in Health Care," *Regulating Health Facilities Construction*, Clark C. Havighurst, ed. (Washington, D.C.: American Enterprise Institute, 1974), p. 268.

That statement put me on record fairly early as subscribing to the view which Professor Kessel, with considerable support from Professors Guido Calabresi and Marc Franklin, has subsequently elaborated, namely that it is poor choice of a liability rule rather than the insidious influence of "commercialism" that is largely to blame for our poor experience with post-transfusion hepatitis.[3] I have also had occasion to examine and endorse a special form of strict liability for post-transfusion hepatitis in a somewhat different context, to which I will refer later.

I have very little to add to what I said in 1971 about the antimarket bias that seems to have inspired Professor Titmuss and his many followers. I dealt there with the subject primarily by quoting Robert Solow's comment on the antimarket bias which he also perceived in *The Gift Relationship*. Solow wrote: "There is a slight, rather typically Fabian, authoritarian streak in Titmuss; he seems to believe that ordinary people ought to be happy to have many decisions made for them by professional experts who will, fortunately, often turn out to be moderately well-born Englishmen."[4] My closing comment on that statement was: "I take it that elitism of the kind referred to is not unknown in the world of medicine." My attempt at pregnant understatement was perhaps less successful than Professor Kessel's low-key observation that "the widespread acceptance of Titmuss's conclusion . . . [despite the inadequacies of his proof] is evidence of strong prior beliefs about the deficiencies of commercialism."[5]

Clearly such "prior beliefs" about market mechanisms are a formidable obstacle to designing institutions which will deliver good-quality blood cheaply but they are only part, perhaps the lesser part, of the problem. I think Professor Kessel may have been correct in suggesting that some of the anticommercialism in the blood sector is simulated rather than real and that fastidiousness of the kind Titmuss professes has been adopted as a convenient stance by those whose worldly interests would be served by a shift to an all-voluntary system. Kessel suggested that avoiding tort liability has been the chief object of the medical establishment in the move to stamp out commercialism, but other benefits would also accrue to the so-called nonprofit sector if such a shift should occur. For example, part of the movement toward eliminating commercial influences and reforming the blood industry is intended to assure the nonprofit sector of a reasonable income, probably through use of the mechanisms of cost-reimbursement and internal cross-subsidization—mechanisms that have contributed heavily to our loss of control over health-care costs generally. In any event, it is interesting to see elements of the medical establishment using the prejudices of a Fabian Socialist to support their case.

[3] R. A. Kessel, "Transfused Blood, Serum Hepatitis, and the Coase Theorem," *Journal of Law and Economics*, vol. 17 (October 1974), pp. 265-89; Guido Calabresi and Kenneth C. Bass, "Right Approach, Wrong Implications: A Critique of McKean on Products Liability," *University of Chicago Law Review*, vol. 38 (1970), p. 74; Marc A. Franklin, "Tort Liability for Hepatitis: An Analysis and a Proposal," *Stanford Law Review*, vol. 24 (1972), pp. 439-80.

[4] Robert M. Solow, "Blood and Thunder," *Yale Law Journal*, vol. 80 (1971), p. 1711.

[5] Kessel, "Transfused Blood," p. 271.

Liability Rules

With these preliminary observations out of the way, I will now consider the development of the law on tort liability for hepatitis, arguing that legal rules designed with incentives and what Professor Coase calls "transaction costs" in mind would have greatly alleviated the problems which Professor Titmuss regarded as conclusive proof of the dangers of commercialism. Then I will briefly discuss some of the legal and extralegal efforts being made to solve these problems by eradicating commercialism rather than by using readily available means of rectifying the market's deficiencies.

Non-Fault-Based Theories. Plaintiffs in cases involving post-transfusion hepatitis have uniformly sought to base their claims on legal theories which do not require them to demonstrate the defendant's negligence. Proof of a provider's actual fault in the procurement, testing, or use of blood would be difficult to produce and would raise many thorny questions, such as the extent of a doctor's or hospital's duty to seek low-risk blood. On the other hand, non-fault-based theories, such as breach of warranty of product quality or the more far-reaching notion of what lawyers call "strict liability in tort" would, if adopted, obviate such proof and would greatly increase not only the frequency of success in prosecuting suits but also the number of suits brought, since lawyers are more likely to accept cases involving low evidence-gathering costs and a high probability of success. Although some courts have been receptive to such non-fault-based theories, the legislatures, influenced by the medical establishment, have not been. The result is that the rule of strict liability has prevailed in no jurisdiction long enough for us to evaluate its impact. The rule of caveat emptor—"let the buyer beware"—has been universally embraced for this product even though that rule is often regarded as an anachronism and has been substantially eroded for many products less hazardous than blood.

Let me now relate some of the developments in this relatively active field, beginning with the cases on implied warranties, an area of law somewhere between contract and tort—that is, between theories that conceive of legal responsibilities as having consensual origins and those that do not.

Implied warranty. The most influential case in this area of non-fault-based liability has been *Perlmutter* v. *Beth David Hospital*, decided by the New York Court of Appeals in 1954.[6] In that case, the plaintiff alleged that the defendant nonprofit hospital had sold her the transfused blood and that therefore implied warranties of fitness and merchantability were applicable to the transaction. The court denied recovery on the theory that there had been no "sale" to which an implied warranty could attach. A distinction between the sale of goods and the

---

[6] Perlmutter v. Beth David Hospital, 308 N.Y. 100, 123 N.E.2d 792 (1954).

provision of services had previously developed in the law of warranties, and the court reasoned that the patient-hospital contract was essentially one for services. The court's conclusion was colored by its recognition that there existed no method for eliminating infected blood.

Courts in many other states have subsequently adopted the rationale of *Perlmutter* whether the defendants were profit making or charitable, hospitals or blood banks.[7] Legal scholars have frequently criticized the decision for its failure to recognize that a sale did in fact take place and, more important, for its reliance on a sales-service dichotomy that no longer reflects the law in many jurisdictions, including New York. Many states now recognize that warranties of fitness and merchantability may arise in nonsales transactions. In spite of wide recognition of these infirmities, the desire to eliminate the implied warranty cause of action for this particular product has generally won out, even though the trend in products-liability law generally has been toward expanding the supplier's responsibility.[8] In 1975, at least two additional states explicitly adopted the *Perlmutter* rationale.[9]

Courts in two states, Illinois and Florida, however, have rejected *Perlmutter* and have characterized blood transfusions as sales rather than services, paving the way for recovery on a non-fault-based theory.[10] Courts in Pennsylvania and New Jersey, on the other hand, have rejected the relevance of the sales-service distinction altogether and have held that, even as a service, a transfusion would give rise to liability on an implied warranty theory.[11] Although the explicit holding in the Pennsylvania case—that a recovery may be possible regardless whether the transfusion is called a sale or a service—has solid support in the law of implied warranties, the decision is apparently not now followed with respect to blood in any jurisdiction. In Pennsylvania and elsewhere, the question has been resolved more or less clearly by legislation precluding recovery on warranty theories of any kind.

Strict liability in tort. In addition to the warranty theory, lawyers can assert an even more novel doctrine, that of strict liability in tort. In the 1970 case of *Cunningham* v. *MacNeal Memorial Hospital*, the Illinois Supreme Court applied

---

[7] See Note, "Strict Liability—The Medical Service Immunity and Blood Transfusions in California," *University of California, Davis, Law Review*, vol. 7 (1974), p. 198, and Franklin, "Tort Liability for Hepatitis," p. 458.

[8] See Note, "Torts—Strict Liability," *Vanderbilt Law Review*, vol. 24 (1970), p. 646 and sources cited therein.

[9] Foster v. Memorial Hospital Association of Charleston, 219 S.E.2d 916 (West Virginia Supreme Court App. 1975); St. Luke's Hospital v. Schmaltz, 534 P.2d 781 (Colo. 1975).

[10] Cunningham v. MacNeal Memorial Hospital, 47 Ill.2d 433, 266 N.E.2d 897 (1970); Russel v. Community Blood Bank, Inc., 185 So.2d 749 (Florida District Court of Appeals, 1966), *affirmed as modified*, 196 So.2d 115 (Florida, 1967).

[11] Hoffman v. Misericordia Hospital, 439 Pa.501, 267 A.2d 867 (1970); Jackson v. Muhlenberg Hospital, 96 N. J. Super. 314, 232 A.2d 879 (1967), *reversed on other grounds*, 53 N.J. 138, 249 A.2d 65 (1969).

this theory and held a hospital strictly liable for hepatitis following a blood trans-fusion regardless of the outcome under the law of warranty.[12] The theory under-lying the doctrine of strict liability in tort is partly that the manufacturer/producer is better able to bear the burden of loss arising from defective products than is the consumer; the victim of the defect is spared catastrophic loss and the burden of his injury is passed on through insurance and higher prices. But, perhaps more important, such liability also stimulates attempts to improve the quality and safety of the product. Over the past thirty years the courts have applied the doctrine of strict liability in tort to an increasingly broad range of products and activities—beginning with abnormally dangerous activities, then including defective foodstuffs and articles for intimate bodily use, and finally encompassing products of all types whether or not manufactured.[13]

Both the plaintiff and the court in the *Cunningham* case relied on the formulation of the doctrine of strict liability in tort adopted in 1965 by the American Law Institute in its *Restatement (Second) of Torts*. The *Restatement*, which is authoritative only in a scholarly sense but is widely relied upon never-theless, states the recommended legal rule at section 402A as follows:

> One who sells any product in a defective condition unreasonably dangerous to the user or consumer or to his property is subject to liability for physical harm thereby caused to the ultimate user or consumer, or to his property, if
> (a) the seller is engaged in the business of selling such a product, and
> (b) it is expected and does reach the user or consumer without substantial change in the condition in which it is sold.[14]

Liability is imposed in spite of the exercise of all possible care and the lack of any contractual relation between the parties.

In the *Cunningham* case the Illinois court found that blood is a "product" within the meaning of section 402A, that the product had been "sold" (rejecting the rationale of *Perlmutter*), and that the blood was "in a defective condition unreasonably dangerous to the user." The defendant hospital contended that transfused blood was "unavoidably unsafe" and therefore fell within an exception to the general rule under the recognized doctrine that some inherently dangerous products (such as pharmaceuticals, with their potential for side effects) are so valuable to society that they should be marketed without fear of liability except for negligence. The court rejected this argument on the theory that the exception could not apply to "impure" products such as infected blood.

The refusal of the Illinois court to apply the exception for "unavoidably

---

[12] Cunningham v. MacNeal Memorial Hospital, 47 Ill.2d 433, N.E.2d 897 (1970).
[13] See footnote 8.
[14] American Law Institute, *Restatement (Second) of Torts* §402A(1) (St. Paul: American Law Institute Publishers, 1965).

unsafe" products and its invention of a purity requirement have been criticized.[15] It appears that only one other court has adopted the *Cunningham* rationale, but its ruling only applies to transfusions predating the 1971 state statute that limited liability.[16] Within the past year, courts in both New York and New Jersey have applied the exception for unavoidably unsafe products under section 402A to blood.[17] The Illinois legislature manifested its disapproval of the *Cunningham* result by eliminating strict liability in tort as a cause of action in transfusion cases. Even if they were inclined to follow *Cunningham*, the great majority of other state courts would probably be precluded from doing so by statutes which prohibit the characterization of blood transfusions as a sale.

Statutory Limitations on Liability. In 1965 only three states had statutes limiting liability for transfusion-related injuries. But as soon as the threat of strict liability was recognized, hospital associations, blood bank groups, and physicians' organizations began successful lobbying campaigns to limit liability to negligence. The political power of these groups stands in marked contrast to the organizational vacuum on the side of potential hepatitis victims, and thus, by 1975, forty-five states had enacted legislation designed to preclude liability of blood suppliers except where negligence was proved.[18] In 1974 Professor Kessel wrote that as a practical matter "strict liability in tort for blood does not exist in the United States. In the states in which legislatures have not granted exemptions to the medical establishment, they have not been needed. . . ."[19] This appears to be an accurate statement. Although frustrated plaintiffs have challenged the constitutionality of these statutes, they have always lost.[20]

The statutes do not provide completely uniform protection for potential defendants. The earlier statutes seeking to codify *Perlmutter* provided only that the procurement, distribution, or use of blood for transfusion purposes did not constitute a sale. A court could avoid this limitation by holding that implied warranties arise in nonsale—that is, service—transactions. But, when the Pennsylvania Supreme Court adopted this approach, the legislature was quick to seal off

---

[15] See Brody v. Overlook Hospital, 127 N. J. Super. 331, 317 A.2d 392 (1974) at 397 for a list of pertinent commentary.

[16] Reilly v. King County Central Blood Bank, Inc., 492 P.2d 246 (Washington App. 1971).

[17] Steinik v. Doctors Hospital, 368 N. Y. S.2d 767 (N. Y. Supreme Court 1975); Brody v. Overlook Hospital, 66 N. J. 448, 332 A.2d 596 (1975); McMichael v. American Red Cross, 532 S. W.2d 7 (Kentucky Court of Appeals, 1975).

[18] For a list of state statutes, see Note, "Blood Transfusions and the Transmission of Serum Hepatitis: The Need for Statutory Reform," *American University Law Review*, vol. 24 (1975), pp. 404-5.

[19] Kessel, "Transfused Blood," p. 278.

[20] See, for example, Glass v. Ingalls Memorial Hospital, 336 N.E.2d 495 (Ill. App. Court, 1975); McKinstrie v. Henry Ford Hospital, 223 N.W.2d 114 (Michigan Court of Appeals, 1974); Bartholomew v. Quakertown Hospital Association, Docket No. 73-9137-08-2 (Pennsylvania Court Comm. Pleas, April 1974).

this route.[21] In two California appellate court cases, plaintiffs lost on their argument that California should imply warranties in transfusion-related "service" transactions.[22] It appears that as of mid-1976 no other state had adopted the rationale of the Pennsylvania Supreme Court.

The second generation of statutes stipulated that no implied warranties were to arise from procurement, distribution, or use of blood regardless of characterization as sale or service. This type of statute does not necessarily block the application of strict liability in tort—since it addresses only the warranty issue—unless the statute is read as also prohibiting characterization of the blood transfer as a sale giving rise to strict liability under the *Restatement* formulation.[23] Even this last hurdle could be surmounted, however, if a court decided to ignore the *Restatement* sale requirement. California courts, for example, have declined to respect the sale requirement of section 402A in other contexts and have decided cases as if it did not exist. Although the California judiciary has so far declined to extend strict liability in tort to transfusion-related injuries, citing precedents of questionable relevance, the California Supreme Court, which has led the way in expanding the scope of products liability, has not yet ruled on these issues.[24]

In spite of the possible loopholes in the statutes, there is now no discernible movement anywhere toward the application of strict liability in tort in blood-transfusion cases. The most recent statutes commonly provide that blood transfers "shall not give rise to any implied warranties of any type and the doctrine of strict tort liability shall not be applicable to the transmission of hepatitis. . . ." At least five states have statutes of this type,[25] and others would probably adopt them if their courts should make it necessary. Probably the courts will recognize the fruitlessness of defying the medical lobby on this point and will not need to be corrected in the future. Indeed, since 1973 all ambiguities have been resolved in favor of defendants. As a practical matter, plaintiffs are now limited to actions based on negligence.

Negligence. Plaintiffs have based their claims on negligence only as a last resort, and only recently have they even bothered to allege it. Few such cases have ever gone to a jury, and, as far as can be told, no court-ordered recovery has yet been obtained. This lack of success in proving negligence does not appear, however, to be the result of a lack of plausible arguments. Rather, the courts have, for policy reasons, declined to analyze carefully the myriad due-care issues that arise.[26]

---

[21] Hoffman v. Misericordia Hospital, 439 Pa. 501, 267 A.2d 867 (1970).

[22] See Note, "Blood Transfusions in California," pp. 201-17.

[23] See for example, McDaniel v. Baptist Memorial Hospital, 469 F.2d 230 (Sixth Circuit, 1972) (applying Tennessee law).

[24] "Blood Transfusions in California," pp. 204-7.

[25] The five are Hawaii, Montana, New Hampshire, New Mexico, and Washington.

[26] Franklin, "Tort Liability for Hepatitis," pp. 446-56 discusses potential negligence issues at length.

The courts have refused to become involved in challenges to a physician's judgment, but the issues that might arise if the courts changed their position include: Was a transfusion really necessary? Is there a duty to use volunteer blood whenever it is available? Is there a duty to use volunteer blood for elective surgery or for older patients? Is there a duty to inform the elective patient that he can wait until volunteer blood is available?

Potential hospital-negligence liability turns on the hospital's use of alternative sources of blood. Must use of allegedly safer volunteer blood always be maximized? Is use of a commercial blood bank negligence per se when volunteer blood is available? In the few cases in point, either these and related questions have been answered in the negative or the court has found adherence to the published standards of the Food and Drug Administration, the American Association of Blood Banks, and the Red Cross to be sufficient to constitute due care.

Professor Franklin has suggested that blood banks could be held liable for lax questioning of donors, for failure to perform adequate tests, for reuse of a donor whose blood had previously been used as part of a multiunit transfusion that resulted in hepatitis, or even for conducting collection operations in high-risk slum areas.[27]

Although the courts may, in reaction to the recent malpractice crisis, continue to be hard to convince of negligence in hepatitis cases, there would seem to be many fruitful lines of argument for plaintiffs' lawyers to pursue.

How a Different Liability Rule Would Make A Difference

With the legal developments before us, we can now ask whether there has not been a serious mistake. Although the legislatures have spoken with remarkable unanimity on the issue of post-transfusion hepatitis, the question may still be debatable. For one thing, no-fault approaches to medical malpractice problems are being actively considered, and this issue is closely related to that debate. Moreover, the final decision on how our blood procurement system is to operate has not been made, and the liability issue may yet come up for further discussion. Finally, it seems unnecessary to regard the state legislatures' judgments on this question as a clear expression of the will of the people, since the case seems to have been a powerful illustration of how an industry can have its way with the legislature when it rallies behind a particular measure and no member of the public perceives himself clearly enough as a potential victim of the measure to oppose it. Thus, there has been no lobbying organization of future victims of post-transfusion hepatitis to contest the views of the medical establishment on the liability question, and plaintiffs' lawyers have lacked a sufficient stake or have been insufficiently persuasive to protect their future clients' interests. It appears that the courts, which

---

[27] Ibid., pp. 447-49.

on several occasions rejected the caveat-emptor position, may have been better placed to look out for the public's welfare than its elected representatives.

Strict liability for post-transfusion hepatitis is called for on a variety of grounds. For one thing, the consequences of a serious illness, the cost of which, according to Kessel, averages $23,000 per episode,[28] can be readily spread by this means from the individual victims to society as a whole. This may be regarded as an important welfare measure in itself, as merely a persuasive argument which justifies the cost of shifting the burden only when cumulated with other arguments, or simply as a makeweight, an attractive feature which makes the thrust of other more powerful arguments more acceptable. (I lean toward this last view.) Another piece of the argument is that a strict rule is relatively easy to administer and, once established, would probably occasion little litigation, producing settlements instead. But the essential argument, which I regard as more than sufficient to tip the balance all by itself, is the creation of incentives for safety. Such incentives, because of consumer ignorance and Professor Coase's transaction costs,[29] are seriously inadequate under a system of caveat emptor for this particular product.

The ways in which the risks of poor-quality blood can be or might be minimized are so numerous and varied that I consider it highly unlikely that any centrally controlled system could possibly find the optimal combination of strategies. Centralized systems are dependent for the fostering of innovations and quality improvements on the competence and good intentions of their managers, who may be chosen for other qualities. Such managers might be counted on, or compelled, to take the obvious steps, but the correct solutions are unlikely to be obvious. For example, the possibilities go far beyond relying solely on donated blood, the preferred strategy at the moment. This strategy is wholly untested as an exclusive production technique in this country, and the costs of pursuing it are largely unknown. Moreover, its adoption requires the destruction of many existing blood-collection systems, and these could turn out, especially under restructured incentives, to be capable of producing a good product more reliably and inexpensively than a centralized system.

No one disputes that donated blood is safer on the average than purchased blood, but averages tell us very little. For one thing, they submerge all the many and possibly important gradations between the perfect, but apparently rare, altruism endorsed by Titmuss on the one hand and purchase for a straight cash payment on the other. For another thing, some purchased blood is apparently quite safe.[30] This fact strongly suggests that the introduction of a liability risk could indeed

---

[28] Kessel, "Transfused Blood," p. 271.

[29] R. H. Coase, "The Problem of Social Cost," *Journal of Law and Economics*, vol. 3 (1960), pp. 1-44.

[30] See, for example, P. W. Holley, G. C. Glenn, and B. Y. Linkerhoker, "Do Volunteer Donors Decrease Post-Transfusion Hepatitis?" *Journal of the American Medical Association*, vol. 234 (December 8, 1975), pp. 1051-52, suggesting that careful selection of donors, rather than reliance on volunteers, should be emphasized in the interest of maximum safety.

substantially improve blood quality without necessarily reducing the quantity of purchased blood consumed. Indeed, the quantity of purchased blood might well increase once its quality had improved enough to remove the current stigma.

Consider the variety of blood-collection strategies available to a blood bank which had an economic motive for avoiding contaminated blood: the location of its collection centers could be changed; donors could be better screened, with longer histories and more searching questions; efforts could focus on a small number of dependable regular donors as opposed to a larger, more erratic group of casual donors; a register of donors could be kept to eliminate those who have shown up as carriers or have been implicated (once or more than once) in a hepatitis incident; payments might vary depending on the donor's progress in establishing his safety; collections from groups such as college students or employees of a given establishment might be emphasized; the medical or work records of such groups might be scrutinized; or, to reduce private incentives to lie, church groups or clubs might be encouraged to use blood donations as a fund-raising technique. Surely other ways might also be thought of by competing blood banks intent on producing a high-quality product without incurring costs which purchasers were unwilling to pay. Note that the choice of a mix of strategies and of the priority to be placed on each involves a trade-off between cost and quality which a centrally directed system could not reliably make but with which competitive markets are usually able to deal very well.

Even if it were clear that the all-volunteer strategy was the cheapest and best way of quickly improving the quality of blood collected, the case for imposing strict liability for post-transfusion hepatitis would still be strong. It is an important insight that the value of incentives for avoiding hepatitis does not stop once reasonably good-quality blood has been procured. As long as any risk remains, providers who are motivated to avoid the costs of this disease will seek cost-effective ways of using blood which minimize the risks still further. Let me list some of the cost-minimization strategies which might be adopted in blood use, again with the purpose of persuading you that the possibilities are so numerous and the choices so unobvious and problematical that we should rely on provider incentives rather than on a centrally managed system to find the optimal solution or set of solutions. Note also that it is asking a good deal of the courts to expect them to enforce efficient behavior by applying their theories of negligence to providers' conduct in these complex matters.

First, providers can use blood components, which are safer than whole blood, in many circumstances, and they might be more willing to do so if they had reason to recognize the potential cost of a hepatitis reaction discounted for the risk involved in the particular case. Since the condition of the individual patient and the quality of the particular whole blood available are factors in the benefit-cost assessment here, there is no easy way to make a regulation dictating the proper decision in every case. But with the right incentives, providers could be expected to make judgments that were in society's interest. Since the risk associated with each unit of blood may be different, it would be desirable for providers to take that factor into account, using higher-risk blood for lower-risk patients. Without the incentive that strict liability provides, however, providers might prefer to rely on a random or first-come, first-served allocation system, leaving hepatitis to chance but allowing it to do more damage when it occurred.

Second, there are tests that can be used to screen the blood itself, but the decision whether they are worth the cost (about $5 per unit for the radioimmuno-assay, as I understand it) depends on the quality of the blood (tried versus untried donors, and so on) and the condition of the patient (young or old, immune or not, and so forth). Also, the incentive provided for the development of better tests would perhaps be a more reliable stimulus to research than those that already exist (though it would be hard to show that there has been underinvestment in blood-related research in the past). Again, centralized decision making, reliance on professional norms, and judicial cost-benefit analyses all seem likely to produce less than the best attainable performance.

Third, decisions whether to use blood at all would be made with greater regard to hepatitis risks if liability were properly assigned. Surgeons would be less inclined than they now are to use blood to achieve a postoperative cosmetic effect—that is, to restore color to the patient's cheeks. The quantity of blood given might be reduced by extending the "one-pint rule" (that is, if all the patient needs is one pint, he does not need blood at all) to call for one pint less than you think the patient needs. Although I would not be so bold as to suggest that shifting the risk of hepatitis would make a dent in the problem of unnecessary surgery, neither would I rule out the possibility that surgeons or hospital tissue-review and utilization-review committees would be marginally more careful if the intro-duction of this new cost slightly altered the expected profitability of each operation. Again, I see great advantages in getting incentives in order so that they can impose a new control, closely coinciding with professional obligations and supplementing the uneven and frequently ineffective professional controls.

Although I said earlier that the rule of strict liability has prevailed nowhere long enough for us to evaluate its effect, after completing the text of this paper I found forgotten in my files a small but I think striking piece of empirical evidence that may persuade this audience (perhaps impatient with my theorizing about the incentive value of strict liability) to take my argument a bit more seriously. The evidence is particularly significant in that it comes from a physician and addresses the crucial question of the relative merit of legally created incentives on the one hand and, on the other hand, the various kinds of quality-promoting activities which the medical profession normally holds out as a fully adequate substitute for more direct regulatory or legal controls on medical practice. This testimonial to the value of incentives appears in a letter to the editor of the *Journal of the*

American Medical Association from a doctor in an Illinois hospital. I will quote it in full since it is not very long:

> Court decisions of medicolegal cases, in general, have resulted in a great influence on the quality of a patient's care. In the field of blood banking, an impact by a medicolegal case has been no exception to this. In the Cunningham case in October, 1970, a hospital was held strictly liable to a patient who allegedly contracted hepatitis after a blood transfusion. This has had national repercussions. The impact has been especially great on our hospital, a 675-bed general hospital, located within 20 miles of the hospital in which the case took place. In view of this, a study was made to evaluate the scope and extent of the effects of the case on blood usage in our hospital.
>
> The study included assessment of 341 charts of patients who received single-unit transfusions in the past three years. In addition, data were collected from the records of the blood bank from 1960 through 1971. There was a significant change in the trends of blood usage between the periods before and after the court decisions. The use of packed cells substantially increased in 1971 ($X^2 = 5.26$; $P<.025$). A significant increase of "necessary" single-unit transfusions was seen in 1971 ($X^2 = 4.12$; $P<.05$). "Unnecessary" transfusions, on the other hand, declined markedly in 1971 ($X^2 = 4.64$; $P<.05$). The general trend of a steady decrease in the number of single-unit transfusions was observed in the last 11 years, but the most recent years showed no significant departure from the trend. Interestingly, a gradual increase in two-unit transfusions was seen in the last seven years, although the increase in the recent years was not statistically significant.
>
> Many approaches to proper use of blood have appeared in literature. [Footnotes omitted.] Almost all of the reports have dealt with the necessity of educational programs for medical staff, establishing a blood bank committee in a hospital, evaluating single-unit transfusions, or establishing a hepatitis follow-up system of patients who received blood. There were, however, very few reports delineating which factors played the most effective role in improving blood usage or the extent of the effects after implementing the proposed program. As a part of educational programs for the medical staff in our hospital, we have regularly issued a news bulletin in the past four years. At the end of 1969, a blood bank committee was set up in our hospital, reviewing all single-unit transfusions. At the same time, a hepatitis follow-up system has been established, sending a letter to the physician whose patient received blood transfusions three months previously. Despite these activities, this study showed no significant changes in the trends of blood usage in 1970.
>
> There has been a general feeling among those engaged in blood banking that the trend of blood usage has changed significantly after the court decision. This study appears to substantiate that feeling. The Cunningham case and the repercussions that followed the case have had, directly or indirectly, a great impact on the minds of physicians, and have played a decisive role in the changes of trends of blood usage.

The impact by the case has been far greater than that by various educational activities hitherto taken in our hospital.[31]

I think Dr. Okuno's letter speaks for itself and for the proposition that the correct liability rule yields benefits which are otherwise practically unattainable. I wish we had evidence not only on blood use but also on the quality of blood collected. I am sure we would find important benefits there as well.

I have dwelt heavily on the value of incentives precisely because it seems inadequate merely to mention them in passing. For example, I find two scholars who reject the strict-liability rule without giving any sign that they appreciate the value of incentives in these circumstances. One, Professor Richard Epstein of the University of Chicago Law School, who touches on the blood problem only superficially in the course of his discussion of a much bigger issue, seems to think that incentives are considered valuable here only because they stimulate research, which is, of course, the smallest part of the argument.[32] The other, Professor Kenneth Fraundorf, in discussing "competition in blood banking," cites Professor Kessel and the issues he raises only in two footnotes.[33] He seems to think that Kessel's argument is simply that liability will in time educate the doctors, who will learn by trial and error from the disasters that befall their patients. My guess is that Kessel's article appeared after Fraundorf's was completed and after Fraundorf was committed to his conclusion that consumer ignorance about hepatitis risks makes a competitive market a dangerous means of producing and allocating blood. He seems to have missed both Calabresi's and Franklin's earlier writing. He also ignores the entire point that liability rules imposing the costs of mistakes on the purveyors of goods can serve as a satisfactory substitute for the consumer's direct knowledge of risks by enlisting producers to act on the consumer's behalf in attempting to avoid injuries. Fraundorf's conclusion about the inadequacy of the market is thus, like Titmuss's, in no way justified by the analysis.

Despite these two dissenters, the weight of scholarly authority is distinctly on the side of strict liability for post-transfusion hepatitis. To the works already cited I can add a piece by Dr. Laurence Tancredi and myself in which we examined post-transfusion hepatitis as a candidate for compensation under a no-fault insurance system which we were attempting to design for dealing with the broader problems of malpractice lawsuits and malpractice itself.[34] I have lately elaborated the no-fault proposal further, defending the need for improved incen-

[31] Takashi Okuno, "The Cunningham Case and Blood Usage," *Journal of the American Medical Association*, vol. 220 (1972), p. 1015.

[32] Richard A. Epstein, "Medical Malpractice: The Case for Contract," *American Bar Foundation Research Journal*, vol. 1976, pp. 116-19.

[33] Kenneth C. Fraundorf, "Competition in Blood Banking," *Public Policy*, vol. 23 (1975), p. 222, n. 5 and p. 228, n. 21.

[34] Clark C. Havighurst and Laurence R. Tancredi," Medical Adversity Insurance—A No-Fault Approach to Medical Malpractice and Quality Assurance," *Milbank Memorial Fund Quarterly: Health and Society*, vol. 51 (1973), pp. 125-64.

tives in medical practice more fully than I have been able to do here.[35] It is important to underscore, however, my strong belief that such incentives are better supplied by a carefully tailored statutory obligation to secure experience-rated insurance protecting patients against clearly defined, largely avoidable hazards than by the vagaries of judicial rule making.

One final issue on which Professor Kessel differs with the other leading students of the question is in naming the physician as the party on whom liability should fall. Calabresi and Bass, Franklin, and Tancredi and I all selected the hospital and the blood bank as the proper risk bearers. Taking a page directly from Professor Coase, however, the Havighurst-Tancredi paper suggests that it really does not make much difference whether the hospital or the doctor is held liable since transactions between them are relatively cheap. Thus, as we put it, "[b]argaining between them would surely be initiated whichever way the responsibility was initially assigned, and it is probable that the same preventive actions would be taken whichever party bore the initial loss."[36]

Legal and Extralegal Moves toward Ensuring a Supply of High-Quality Blood

Let me now discuss briefly the steps currently being taken to deal with the problem of blood quality. It appears that almost all these steps build on a premise which I believe I have shown to be shaky—namely, that there is no way of rehabilitating the market for purchased blood to improve product quality and that therefore the market must be altered and "commercial" influences eliminated.

There is also underway a movement to substitute central control for market forces as the primary allocative mechanism through a system of "regionalization." Professor Fraundorf's article argues that the market mechanism would work quite well for distributing blood and avoiding waste through outdating if commercial banks were permitted to function freely.[37] He contends that these for-profit firms could be counted on to engage in arbitrage, adjusting marginal imbalances in supply and demand in a way that nonprofit banks apparently do not. It appears, therefore, that it is still the problem of blood quality that supplies the leading objective argument for the changes being considered.[38]

---

[35] Clark C. Havighurst, "Medical Adversity Insurance—Has Its Time Come?" *Duke Law Journal*, vol. 1975, pp. 1233-80.

[36] Havighurst and Tancredi, "Medical Adversity Insurance," p. 146, n. 6. This a direct application of the "Coase theorem." See Coase, "The Problem of Social Cost."

[37] Fraundorf, "Competition in Blood Banking," pp. 219-40.

[38] There is also an argument that people who would give blood will not take money for it and that people are less willing to donate blood when it can be sold. This argument raises empirical issues, not about whether the assertions are true but about which system is capable of better performance in terms of quality, quantity, and cost. Subjective preferences might not yield to such empirical evidence, but presumably such preferences should ultimately be expressed by legislatures, which might be more impressed by considerations of efficiency.

Legal Discrimination between Commercial and Nonprofit Suppliers. A few states have imposed special burdens on commercial blood banks. Thus, an Idaho statute allows a damage suit for post-transfusion hepatitis to be brought on a strict-liability theory only against for-profit blood banks or in cases where the donor was compensated.[39] Similarly, the state of Washington makes an exception to its general proscription of actions based on strict liability theories for "any trans-action in which the blood donor receives compensation."[40] These statutes have not been tested in court to see if the classifications they establish are constitutionally reasonable. The evidence cited by Kessel that some purchased blood is of reasonable quality suggests that they may not be.

The Wisconsin Supreme Court has overturned a state statutory prohibition against the operation of for-profit blood banks on the ground that it imposed an impermissible burden on interstate commerce.[41] The Idaho and Washington statutes might be subject to similar objections, among others.

Labeling Blood as Donated or Purchased. A seemingly less Draconian measure than the foregoing is the introduction of a labeling requirement that allows providers and consumers to distinguish between donated and purchased blood. Illinois was the first state to adopt such a measure, and California has recently followed suit.[42] The Food and Drug Administration proposed regulations in November 1975 to introduce such a requirement at the federal level, but this proposal has attracted some opposition, most notably from the Council on Wage and Price Stability.[43] The rules are not yet final. The FDA proposal would also require that each package include a warning that paid-donor blood is associated with a higher hepatitis risk.

Proponents of this strategy present it as a full disclosure requirement. But the possibility exists that the required disclosure involves only a half-truth in that it tends to present all paid-donor blood as equally risky and all donated blood as safer than all purchased blood. As I have suggested, this is not necessarily the whole story.

One might argue, of course, that consumers are simply put on reasonable notice of a real risk and could still elect to purchase the commercially procured product because of either a lower price or some additional information about the quality of the particular commercial source. Normally this would be a persuasive argument, but for the blood market it is too simple because there are reasons to

---

[39] Idaho Code §39-3702 (Supp. 1975).

[40] Rev. Code Wash. Ann. §70.54.120 (1975).

[41] The State of Wisconsin v. Interstate Blood Bank, Inc., 65 Wis.2d 482, 222 N.W.2d 912 (1974).

[42] Ill. Ann. Stat. tit. 91 §182 (Smith-Hurd Supp. 1974); California Health and Safety Code §1603.5 (West 1976). See "California Mandates Blood Labeling," *Medical World News*, November 3, 1975, pp. 46-47.

[43] 40 Fed. Reg. 53040 (November 1975).

think that the consumer's agents charged with making blood-purchasing decisions are excessively disinclined to consider cost, to seek out additional quality information, and to act on such information even when they have it. Thus, doctors and hospitals may attach excessive importance to the mandated labels out of a fear of malpractice suits. Even if they have good reasons for using commercial blood, the safest defensive posture is to avoid having to offer explanations before a jury. Thus, the professional tendency to practice "defensive medicine," much criticized when it suits the profession and others to discredit the tort system, is being relied upon by proponents of labeling measures to generate a bias against commercial blood suppliers, even those whose product may be of satisfactory quality.

In view of these considerations, it seems to me that the Illinois and California laws and the FDA proposal involve overkill of the paid donor and serve primarily the narrow interests of the nonprofit sector.

National Blood Policy and the American Blood Commission. The remaining responses to the problem of poor-quality blood fall somewhat outside my assigned topic since they are not, strictly speaking, legal responses. I am not prepared to characterize them as *il*legal, though I have some questions in this regard, but they are certainly extralegal, being the product of gratuitous action by the federal bureaucracy and private initiatives responding thereto. I refer, of course, to the so-called National Blood Policy and the attempts of the American Blood Commission to implement it. As I understand it, the National Blood Policy was conceived by the Department of Health, Education, and Welfare at the request of the President but without any specific statutory mandate and the American Blood Commission has no legal standing beyond that supplied by HEW's approval.

In particular, the American Blood Commission has no warrant to take steps offensive to the antitrust laws and would be treated for antitrust purposes like any other private association that set out to reform an industry by private agreements. Since I do not know precisely what the commission proposes to do, I am unable to express an opinion on the antitrust aspects of its activities. I do understand, however, that the Antitrust Division of the Department of Justice is aware of its existence, and it may be that the division can be induced to take a tolerant view of what it does. I am not persuaded, however, that antitrust principles should be relaxed to allow the attainment of the Blood Commission's worthy purposes. It would be better, I think, to put the question in the hands of Congress for a definitive decision one way or the other on the nation's future blood policy.

Whether or not the Antitrust Division should bless the commission's plans to regionalize the blood industry and curtail the role of commercial blood banks, the commission may well feel that it needs an antitrust exemption from Congress to accomplish its purposes without undue exposure to private antitrust actions. Such an exemption has been proposed in the past, primarily to permit nonprofit blood banks, physicians, and hospitals to engage in concerted refusals to deal with particular blood suppliers which would otherwise be per se violations of the Sherman Act.[44]

In debating the case for allowing the American Blood Commission to engage in such restraints or others, Congress would have the opportunity to examine the alternative strategy of restructuring incentives in the blood market, an alternative which, I have argued, has had an insufficient hearing and which I believe is at least as likely as the American Blood Commission to ensure a dependable supply of good-quality blood at reasonable cost. For this reason, I would urge the Antitrust Division to do nothing that might reduce the necessity for the American Blood Commission to seek explicit antitrust exemptions before taking questionable steps to carry out the National Blood Policy. I would hope that Congress, in considering a proposal for such an exemption, would also give explicit consideration to a bill proposing the reintroduction of a kind of strict liability for post-transfusion hepatitis, perhaps, as Franklin has suggested, by requiring hospitals to provide, at their own expense, experience-rated insurance protection for patients who receive transfusions. Perhaps, before acting on such a proposal, Congress (or HEW) could undertake to test the conflicting hypotheses by approving a major experiment with such insurance in an area having a large number of commercial blood suppliers.

In my view, the reintroduction of strict liability (through insurance) would be appropriate whether or not an antitrust exemption were granted to permit the elimination of commercial blood suppliers. Such insurance, if properly priced, would induce closer attention to the correct use of blood in therapy and additional care in blood procurement. It would also be a desirable way of maintaining accountability for the results of medical treatment and would serve to advance the cause of a no-fault, incentive-oriented compensation system for other medical injuries, something which is likely to be given serious study.[45] Like Dr. Okuno, I see no other effective way of changing doctors' and hospitals' behavior.

It seems likely that one positive result of this conference will be to make the policy choices available in this industry clearer than they have been heretofore. Of course, the proposal advanced here for a return to a form of strict liability will not be popular with the blood industry itself. But that is not a sufficient reason for Congress to reject it.

---

[44] H.R. 4842, 93rd Congress, 1st session, 1973. See also Community Blood Bank of the Kansas City Area, Inc., No. 8519 (F.T.C., September 28, 1966), *reversed on other grounds*, 405 F.2d 1011 (6th Circuit 1969).

[45] The American Bar Association's Commission on Medical Professional Liability has recommended and is seeking funds for a study of "medical adversity insurance," perhaps leading to a pilot insurance program which could well include post-transfusion hepatitis as a compensable outcome.

BLOOD AND ALTRUISM:
AN ECONOMIC REVIEW

A. J. Culyer

Hamlet has but one prince; the controversy about blood has had two. Alas, neither Richard Titmuss nor Reuben Kessel is with us any more, though the ideas of both will doubtless be our major concern at this conference. We must hope that our discussion will not be like *Hamlet* without the prince, even though we are immeasurably worse off without the benefit of the wisdom of these two men.

I shall take Titmuss as a starting point and consider both of the aspects of the debate as he identified them: on the one hand, the overt issues concerning the best ways of collecting and distributing blood and, on the other, the indirect issues relating to social policy and the role of altruism in society. In the space of a single paper I shall, I fear, do the second of these issues even less justice than I shall do the first.

As is often the case with controversies ultimately involving general but fundamental values and growing out of a specific context of discussion, the literature is marked by lapses into special pleading and by confusion about what precisely is at issue. With hindsight, for example, I believe it is fairly clear that empirical questions have frequently been confused with questions of principle. If, however, we are to maximize the advantages of hindsight, there is much to be said for considering the contexts in which the discussion began and has since developed. Then, perhaps, we can try to cope with the muddles.

The Early Context

The involvement of social scientists in the argument about blood began with a Fabian lecture delivered by Richard Titmuss in 1966 and subsequently published as a Fabian pamphlet.[1] Those were the days, for those of you with memories long enough to recall them, when most economists were happily committing the "grass is greener" fallacy, even thought it had several times been thoroughly exposed by those favoring an explicit comparative analysis of behavior under differing institutional constraints. The fallacy was to suppose that a case for government provision of services could be built merely by observing instances of what at that time was called market "failure." The principal sources to which we referred

---

[1] Richard M. Titmuss, *The Gift Relationship: From Human Blood to Social Policy* (London: Allen and Unwin, 1970).

students in those days were all highly skeptical of the market and of the virtues of competition—even if the AMA's restrictive practices could have been curtailed—in the medical marketplace.[2] In Britain, however, a strong countermovement supporting the market was initiated by Dennis Lees in 1960 and was supported in papers published through the sixties, notably by John and Sylvia Jewkes.[3] Titmuss was by far the most assiduous critic of "economists" (of the Lees-Jewkes variety) in Britain.

Much of the a priori flavor of the argument concerned the logical applicability of the economic paradigm and the applicability of the standard theorems of the so-called new welfare economics. Although I think Titmuss's position at that time was probably not one of total rejection of economics (rather, he would probably have insisted on the necessity of its insights' being complemented and qualified by those of other disciplines—a view to which many of us are sympathetic), much of his writing appeared to be directed at the fundamental question of the applicability of economic theory. The literature of the 1960s typically assumed that a list of "characteristics" of medical care could be drawn up showing that health care was so different from other services that the market could not allocate it efficiently, though, of course, the state could.[4]

It was in this context that Titmuss introduced a question that he clearly thought would sow confusion among the opposition: "is human blood a consumption good?"[5] That Titmuss underestimated the tenacity of the opposition is well enough illustrated by the fact that as recently as 1974 the late Reuben Kessel was able to conclude that the defects of the U.S. blood market were attributable more to the absence of a commercial market than to its presence.

It was primarily to answer the basic question posed by Titmuss that Cooper and Culyer rose to the defense of the economic approach, though not necessarily

---

[2] See for example, Burton A. Weisbrod, *Economics of Public Health* (Philadelphia: University of Pennsylvania Press, 1961); Harold M. Somers and Anne R. Somers, *Doctors, Patients and Health Insurance* (Washington, D.C.: Brookings Institution, 1961); Kenneth J. Arrow, "Uncertainty and the Welfare Economics of Medical Care," *American Economic Review*, vol. 53 (1963); Herbert E. Klarman, *The Economics of Health* (New York: Columbia University Press, 1965).

[3] See Dennis S. Lees, "The Economics of Health Services," *Lloyds Bank Review* (April 1960); idem, "The Logic of the British National Health Service," *Journal of Law and Economics*, vol. 5 (1962); idem (with others), *Monopoly and Choice in Health Services* (London: Institute of Economic Affairs, 1964); idem, "Efficiency in Government Spending: Social Services—Health," *Public Finance*, vol. 22 (1967); idem (with Robert G. Rice), "Uncertainty and the Welfare Economics of Medical Care," *American Economic Review*, vol. 55 (1965); John and Sylvia Jewkes, *The Genesis of the British National Health Service* (Oxford: Basil Blackwell, 1961); idem, *Value for Money in Medicine* (Oxford: Basil Blackwell, 1963).

[4] A critical review of the arguments is in Anthony J. Culyer, "The Nature of the Commodity 'Health Care' and Its Efficient Allocation," *Oxford Economic Papers*, vol. 23 (1971). It is no exaggeration to say that scarcely a health economics reference began in those days without a catalogue of reasons why "health" was "different."

[5] Richard M. Titmuss, *Choice and the Welfare State* (London: Fabian Society, 1967), reprinted in Richard M. Titmuss, *Commitment to Welfare* (London: Allen and Unwin, 1968), p. 147.

to that of the market.[6] The Cooper/Culyer paper was also addressed, albeit indirectly, to another related set of questions concerning the "spheres of influence" of the various social sciences. The paper clearly adhered to the view which holds that economics has a role to play whenever reasonable, articulated objectives can be identified among the members of a society without an abundance of means to achieve those ends; that the divisions of the social sciences are *not* defined by the subject matter they study but by the presumptions they make and the methods they apply; that economic theory is a theory of rational behavior, with both normative and positive implications, rather than a theory of priced, physical, and traded goods. Although the present context is not, perhaps, the right one for a full treatment of the issues this view raises, it is helpful in understanding the form some of the controversy took, for this view was one that Titmuss most certainly did not share. Substantial parts of his book were directed precisely against what has been called "economic imperialism" by those who believe that the disciplines *are* in fact to be distinguished by their subject matter. As observed above, this did not imply that Titmuss viewed the role of economics as negligible but it did imply that he saw the role of economics as different from that perceived by most economists, especially of the younger generation.

Much of the Cooper/Culyer paper amounted to what, in retrospect, is a somewhat tedious exercise in definitions—of "economic good," "free good," "waste," "shortage," "transaction costs," "social costs," and the like. After a brief look at some evidence of shortage and waste in Britain and a statement about the necessary elasticity conditions, the paper concluded that payment in cash or kind would increase supplies of blood but that it might or might not be a less costly way of increasing supplies from the community than advertising or making it more convenient for people to give blood. Moreover, Cooper and Culyer said, for the transfusion service to charge British hospitals a "shadow price" per unit of blood would provide them with an incentive to be efficient.

A deficiency of the Cooper/Culyer paper was its total failure to discuss the problem of serum hepatitis. Instead, two questions were provided in the set of discussion questions at the end: "There is evidence to show that blood from professional donors is more likely to carry disease. What difference does this make to the economic analysis of this *paper?*" and "Is it right to subject patients to additional risks by transfusing them with inferior blood? Compare your answer with the treatment by inferior surgeons, hospitals, etc. If inferiority is a reflection of the fundamental fact of scarcity, can anything be done to remove it?"[7] Unfortunately, again, the answers subsequently given to these questions were not what the authors had expected. For example, Solow (usually a good student!) wrote:

---

[6] Michael H. Cooper and Anthony J. Culyer, *The Price of Blood* (London: Institute of Economic Affairs, 1968).

[7] Ibid., p. 46.

I am afraid I can imagine what [Cooper and Culyer] would find as an acceptable answer to these questions. It would presumably involve the labelling of some blood as "risky" and some as "safe". (Since blood cannot practically be tested for safety, presumably all blood from paid donors would have to be labelled as risky; perhaps one can imagine several grades according to the type of donor—alcoholic, penniless artist, poor but honest, little old lady. But the grade-labelling would have to be policed to avoid cheating, so there is danger of interference with economic liberty even here). Risky blood would of course sell at a lower price than safe blood. Poor people would buy cheap blood; rich people could afford safe blood. If that strikes you as awful, reflect on the fundamental fact of scarcity. Upon reflection, it may not be clear to you that the mere fact of scarcity implies that the quality of blood a man receives should be correlated with his capacity to earn income. You may even be troubled by the fact that the risky blood gets introduced into an otherwise reasonably satisfactory situation only through Cooper and Culyer's belief that buying and selling blood is a useful practice. Suppose that the introduction of a commercial market would in fact result in some marginal improvement in efficiency (though Titmuss's story suggests it wouldn't). The judgment that such an improvement could justify the creation of differentials in quality of blood received by income class does strike me as morally obtuse.[8]

Although other comments have been less restrained,[9] it is clear that the early emphasis on generalities (a common feature of most of the juiciest contributions to the market debate) has encouraged people to infer what they should not. It is particularly ironic that the charge of monotechnism implicit in these criticisms of the original Cooper/Culyer paper (the proposition that the market is the only effective mechanism for collecting blood) should be made against authors who were themselves strongly critical of monotechnism (the proposition that donation is the only effective mechanism for collecting blood). We should point out, however, that Rottenberg does not apparently dissent from Solow's gloss on the implications of differential quality.[10]

The general trend in those days, however, was to write in a rather aggressive and provocative style which probably encouraged the antagonists to see the opposition as a homogeneous camp. Anyone criticizing Titmuss tended to be identified as a dyed-in-the-wool Samuel Smilesian and anyone supporting him was identified as a romantic denier of the existence of scarcity. In the rest of this paper I shall assume that we no longer need these stereotypes and can eschew for good the use of ad hominem arguments.

---

[8] Robert M. Solow, "Blood and Thunder," *Yale Law Journal*, vol. 80 (1971), p. 170.

[9] For example, Mike Reddin, "Economics of Blood and Supply," *Lancet* (May 8, 1971); Anthony J. Culyer, "Ethics and Economics in Blood-Supply," *Lancet* (March 20, 1971); and "Social Scientists and Blood Supply," *Lancet* (June 12, 1971).

[10] Simon Rottenberg, "The Production and Exchange of Used Body Parts," in *Toward Liberty: Essays in Honor of Ludwig von Mises on the Occasion of His 90th Birthday*, vol. 2 (Menlo Park: Institute for Humane Studies, 1971).

So what might Cooper and Culyer have found to be a satisfactory answer to these questions? A good undergraduate might have written, after a cursory trawl through some epidemiological literature:

> There is some probability that any individual blood supplier will be a hepatitis carrier; there is another probability that the carrier's blood (or plasma) will infect a transfused patient; there is another probability that an infected patient will become seriously ill; and there is a final probability that infected patients or their blood will transmit the disease to other patients, hospital staff, and so on.
>
> Each of these probabilities is, of course, dependent upon a variety of variable factors. For example, it seems that some nations and races are more prone to be carriers than others; that drug addicts and prisoners are likewise more prone, as well as those who are generally undernourished. Moreover, those who have a financial incentive to lie about their medical history are more likely to lie and hence have a higher probability of being carriers. In addition, those for whom financial incentives are most likely to be attractive are also those (the poor, drug addicts, and so on) who have higher probabilities.
>
> We know that some carriers, but not all, can be detected. We know that through careful management the other probabilities can be reduced. We know also that none of these probabilities can as yet be reduced to zero. We know also that each method of probability reduction has social costs associated with it. We can infer with reasonable certitude from people's behavior that society is not absolutely risk-averse. Finally, we may further infer from behavior that the social value of good health or even of longer life is not infinite.
>
> If now we also allow that rewarding blood donors will increase the frequency of donation out of a given pool of donors or the size of the pool or both, then society confronts three related sets of choices. The first set relates to choice of the means of procuring a given rate of supply of given quality; the second relates to the preferred quality; the third relates to the preferred quantity. In addition, there may be a choice between rewarding (marginal) donors, with its consequent possible erosion of altruism, and not rewarding them, with its possible consequences in terms of reduced health-giving supplies of blood. There are also subsidiary choices concerning, for example, the preferred maximum frequency with which an individual may supply a unit of his blood. The choice between these will depend upon the value placed upon avoiding risks, whose values are to count, and the costs of avoiding risks and obtaining additional supplies.

This, to my mind, might have been a quite satisfactory undergraduate answer.

In the context of the British National Health Service (NHS) it would manifestly not make a great deal of sense to identify as an implication of the hepatitis risk that patients would pay different prices for different qualities of blood. This part of Solow's answer cannot therefore be regarded as very satisfactory. Indeed, one could plausibly argue the contrary: since equality in ill health is an axiom of the NHS, not only should patients pay no price (as they do now) but they should all receive the same quality blood (good, bad, or indifferent). The main difference for the analysis introduced by the hepatitis risk concerns how, given society's nonabsolute risk-aversion, the risk is best reduced bearing in mind that more resources devoted to that end mean fewer available for other objectives. Given the necessity for this trade-off, who would make it? Presumably the task of social scientists is not to identify the proper arbiters but to explore alternative technologies with their consequential outcomes in terms of costs and benefits to society.

If we were to venture a guess as to what was agreed by everyone at this stage we should reap a relatively poor harvest. Nevertheless, I would venture the following humble assessment: we could probably all agree that much of the argument was less about substantive theoretical and empirical issues than about words. If we accept the broad definition given to "economic good" by virtually all economists, we could agree that blood indeed fell within its scope but that this implies nothing about how, institutionally, it is best procured and distributed. We could probably agree that in principle the choices outlined in the preceding paragraph are, indeed, the choices we confront.

To go further, we need some explicit idea of the objectives of blood procurement in health services, theories of how different institutions may serve those ends and empirical evidence enabling us to discriminate between these alternative theories.

Procedural Options

In *The Gift Relationship* Titmuss could have readily conceded that the dilemmas noted above exist "in principle." In practice, he argued, the evidence shows that the problem of objectives—one is trading-off quality and quantity—is a non-problem because voluntary donation delivers not only the highest quality blood but also more blood per capita than commercial methods. The principal theoretical observations Titmuss made were twofold: namely, (1) that commercialism is inefficient technically because it encourages mendacity and does not lend itself to a rational coordination of blood procurement and distribution to eliminate waste, and (2) that it was inefficient economically for additional reasons related to external costs imposed on the community. Titmuss adopted, of course, a broad notion of efficiency which should find sympathetic ears among contemporary economists. He amassed a large quantity of evidence which seemed to support both his conjecture about the quantity/quality trade-off and the theoretical points about the performance of the two major alternatives, paying individual blood suppliers and selling to hospitals on the one hand and collecting voluntary donations on the other.

A side issue that received scant attention from Titmuss concerns the effects of commercialism in the higher reaches of the "market." Titmuss asserted that the "commercialization of blood and donor relationships . . . sanctions the making of profits in hospitals and clinical laboratories."[11] It is not at all clear to me what this means but I suspect it implies that commercialism in one area "breeds" commercialism in other neighboring areas. If so, examples to the contrary are so abundant as to refute the general implication completely. Surely Titmuss cannot have meant that nonprofit institutions can survive only if they get all their inputs free of charge.

The validity of the evidence related to our main theme has been much debated, though there would seem to be agreement on two points: (1) commercialism provides an incentive for individuals to lie about their health status and (2) hepatitis is more likely to be contracted from blood purchased from the subsets of the population from which it is currently drawn than from blood donated by those who seem, on Titmuss's evidence (in Britain though not in the United States), to be broadly representative of society.

The quantity issue is extremely difficult to settle on the available evidence. Titmuss made much of his observation that blood supplies in Britain have continuously grown while the admittedly patchy evidence for the United States suggested that growth in commercial sources seemed in the 1960s to have been more than offset by a decline in voluntary sources. Evidence on the postponement of operations was, perhaps inevitably, impressionistic, based on quotations from observers who had no systematic evidence.[12] Cooper and Culyer pointed out that the growth of the blood supply in Britain tells us nothing about excess demand.[13] They also introduced evidence that at least some physicians postpone operations because of shortages, and there is plenty of hearsay evidence about regional shortages from time to time or about patients' being given unmatched blood when enough of their own type was not available. Related worries were expressed by Arrow.[14] On balance, however, my own judgment would be that shortages probably have been rather unimportant in Britain. The principal reason for taking this view is one adduced by Titmuss but not given great prominence: the Blood Transfusion Service in England and Wales has never been under any great pressure from hospitals, the medical professions, or patients to rectify severe shortages, and these groups are not famous for their failure to cry "shortage" of anything from the highest available rooftop.[15]

---

[11] Titmuss, *Gift Relationship*, p. 245.

[12] Ibid., pp. 66-67.

[13] Cooper and Culyer, *Price of Blood* and "The Economics of Giving and Selling Blood," in Armen A. Alchian et al., *The Economics of Charity* (London: Institute of Economic Affairs, 1973).

[14] Kenneth J. Arrow, "Gifts and Exchanges," *Philosophy and Public Affairs*, vol. 1 (1972).

[15] Titmuss, *Gift Relationship*, pp. 120-21.

A more interesting question relates, perhaps, to meeting future demand: whether or not future supplies can be increased sufficiently by merely doubling the number of calls made upon existing donors each year, as asserted by Reddin in reply to Culyer, is an empirical matter.[16] Whether this is less costly than some of the alternative methods of obtaining a given increase is again an empirical matter, as is the question whether eliminating money prices to blood suppliers altogether would reduce the U.S. blood supply below current rates or raise costs above current levels. A priori, anything could happen. Empirically we simply do not know.

Titmuss's evidence that a high incidence of hepatitis is necessarily associated with the commercial procurement of blood has also been hotly contested. Cooper and Culyer argued that the incidence of post-transfusion hepatitis depended, in part, on the prevalence of carriers of the antigen in various subgroups of the population.[17] Despite the existence of *homo mendax,* they argued that payment of suppliers drawn from social groups with ostensibly low prevalence rates and payment in forms unlikely to appeal to drug addicts and other groups known to have high prevalence rates would both reduce the incidence of post-transfusion hepatitis. Similar points had and have been made by a number of others.[18]

Most authorities could agree that the following precautions would probably be conducive to a reduction in hepatitis incidence:[19]

(1) Use supplies from socioeconomic groups having a low a priori probability of being antigen carriers.

(2) Test for the presence of the antigen.

(3) Keep the donor pool as small as is consistent with maintaining "adequate" supplies and donor health.

(4) Utilize post-transfusion-hepatitis incidence to eliminate tainted batches.

(5) Do not pool blood "excessively" from different donors or socioeconomic groups.

---

[16] Mike Reddin, "A Dialogue on Blood: 2," *New Society,* March 31, 1975; Anthony J. Culyer, "A Dialogue on Blood: 1," *New Society,* March 24, 1975.

[17] Cooper and Culyer, "Economics of Giving and Selling Blood."

[18] Culyer, "Ethics and Economics"; E. R. Jenning, "Not All Paid Donors Pose Hepatitis Risks," *Laboratory Medicine,* vol. 2 (1971); National Heart and Lung Institute, *Blood Resource Studies,* 1972, appendix C; Thomas R. Ireland and James V. Koch, "Blood and American Social Attitudes," in Alchian et al., *Economics of Charity;* Reuben A. Kessel, "Transfused Blood, Serum Hepatitis, and the Coase Theorem," *Journal of Law and Economics,* vol. 17 (1974); Harvey M. Sapolsky and Stan N. Finkelstein, in "Blood Policy Revisited, *Public Interest,* no. 46 (1977), report a study by the General Accounting Office of paid and unpaid donors which shows that the variance in the number of hepatitis carriers was explained better by socioeconomic factors *other than* whether payment was received.

[19] The first four of these are from Kessel, "Transfused Blood," p. 274.

(6) Ensure the possibility of identifying the source of blood used in transfusion.

(7) Maintain scrupulous cleanliness at all stages of handling blood and managing transfused patients.

(8) Give gamma globulin to all transfused patients.

(9) Give prima facie low-quality blood only to those patients (for example, some hemophiliacs) with known immunity to hepatitis.

(10) Use high prices to produce an excess supply of blood offers or prices-in-kind to select suppliers with low a priori probabilities of carrying the antigen.

Points (1) through (9) apply equally to paid and unpaid systems of collection. Whether such a battery of complementary procedures would reduce the incidence of post-transfusion hepatitis connected with blood from commercial sources to the level believed to be characteristic of blood from unpaid sources is, of course, an empirical question. Whether the risk differential would be "acceptable" to society is not an empirical question, nor is it one, I think, that we are competent to answer since it would require us to make value judgments as to whose preferences are going to "count" in society and what is the proper attitude about risk. So far as I am aware, the techniques of medicine, economics, and sociology can provide us with no answers to these questions. In other words, there may be consumption externalities of the sort that make my utility dependent upon the risks *you* take of contracting hepatitis. But the consequences for an efficient policy depend crucially upon whether these externalities really do exist (a factual matter), what form they take (again a factual matter), whether they should be considered in describing a social optimum, and, if so, whether all forms should be equally worthy of consideration in normative matters.[20]

Institutions

Since I have found no item in the literature which suggests that current U.S. institutional methods for collecting, processing, and distributing blood and its derivatives cannot be made more perfect, I take it that here is another point of agreement. Disagreement is, of course, rife as to how improvements might be made.

Several authors usefully draw on the contemporary economic literature of

---

[20] Titmuss would presumably have paid something (if necessary) to reduce *my* risk. He may also have been prepared to equalize my risk and someone else's, keeping the mean risk the same. Whether these concerns, either or both, are relevant to social welfare is plainly a normative matter, just as is the question of the relevance of another person's willingness to pay to *increase* my risk or to *increase* the variance of risks.

"property rights" or entitlements. Arrow, for example, points out that "The price system, in order to work at all, must involve the concept of property [but] the price system is not, and perhaps in some basic sense cannot be, universal. To the extent that it is incomplete, it must be supplemented by an implicit or explicit social contract."[21] Areas where the price mechanism is highly attenuated include the much-researched area of transactions within the firm and the family. Most of the explanations offered for the absence of a market within these institutions seem to be based upon assumed high costs of transacting. In the health field, Arrow himself suggested that the relatively high costs of private insurance make the health-care market less efficient than universal public insurance.[22] Various kinds of externality argument have also been used to "explain" why the British NHS may be more efficient than the market.[23] Of course, to postulate a more technological objective for health services than is common in the economic literature may also lead to the conclusion that the market is not an appropriate mechanism for distributing these services. For example, to postulate that the objective of health services is to minimize, subject to a resource constraint, the ill health of the community is, while not without its own problems of measurement and value, to postulate such an objective.[24] It is plainly easy to see that the minimization of ill health in the community may more cheaply be accomplished by nonmarket methods—even granted that the market may better satisfy consumer preferences and granted that the market would constitute less of a threat to individual liberty.

Most of these arguments, however, while casting doubt on the usefulness of market prices on the final consumer side of the medical-care industry, scarcely question the usefulness of prices as aids to efficient production. For example, Cooper and Culyer considered paying suppliers of blood and charging hospitals for its use. But they did not (in the context of the British NHS) suggest charging patients.[25]

Rottenberg argues that the market can do a great deal to promote efficiency.

It is true that laboratories cannot screen out blood from hepatitic suppliers. But the market can do so. It is known that the incidence of histories of hepatitis varies with the social class of the suppliers. Since there are gains to be made from keeping separate blood coming from

---

[21] Arrow, "Gifts and Exchanges," p. 357.

[22] Arrow, "Uncertainty and Medical Care." See also Lees and Rice, "Uncertainty and Medical Care," and Kenneth J. Arrow, "Reply," *American Economic Review*, vol. 55 (1965).

[23] For example: Cotton M. Lindsay, "Medical Care and the Economics of Sharing," *Economica*, no. 136 (1969) and Anthony J. Culyer, "Medical Care and the Economics of Giving," *Economica*, no. 151 (1971).

[24] For a development of this view see Anthony J. Culyer, *Need and the National Health Service: Economics and Social Choice* (London: Martin Robertson, 1976).

[25] Cooper and Culyer, *Price of Blood*.

the different social classes, it would not be surprising to discover firms who certify that they have blood taken from subsets of the population in which the incidence of hepatitis is low. . . . we would expect of course, that the market will establish a higher price for high-quality blood and a lower price for low-quality blood. Buyers would be free to choose among the distinguishable classes of blood, taking account of the magnitudes of qualitative difference and the differences in price.[26]

Although he does not say so, Rottenberg would presumably argue that if the demand for high-quality blood is sufficiently great (at the relative price of high-quality blood) the good-quality blood will drive out the bad. Presumably, again, the reason why this has not happened is that either (1) the demand is not sufficiently high, (2) buying blood is not legally permitted, or (3) some combination of these two is the case. So far as I am aware the price paid by hospitals or patients for blood in the United States does not vary according to the a priori quality of the blood.

More generally, it would seem that the essence of the argument about institutions concerns the related property-right issues: who should have the right to what degree of liability for bad blood, and should that liability be tradable? Titmuss argued that the risk to the patient should be at its technological minimum regardless of cost and that the institutional supplier's liability should be total. Titmuss did not specify how this liability should be apportioned or whether it should be tradable or insurable. Rottenberg seems to argue that the supplier's liability should be to provide blood of a stated quality; the consumer then chooses what he prefers. Cooper and Culyer argued implicitly that a public decision is taken about the appropriate quality to be supplied to all customers of the health service. They left open how malpractice and hence legal liability would be defined. Presumably, if the recommended procedures had not been followed by the Blood Transfusion Service and by the relevant hospitals and doctors in a case of post-transfusion hepatitis, then there would be a prima facie case of malpractice.

Kessel, however, has explored the property-right issue more explicitly than any other writer.[27] His argument is related to his earlier theme of medical monopoly.[28] Essentially, the argument is that in the United States the risk has been borne by the patient because it is in the self-interest of organized medicine, the hospitals, and the blood banks to oppose transference of liability from the patient to the institutional suppliers.[29] He argued that charitable blood banks and the American Red Cross oppose strict liability because this would require them

---

[26] Rottenberg, "Production and Exchange of Used Body Parts," pp. 330-31.

[27] Kessel, "Transfused Blood, Serum Hepatitis, and the Coase Theorem."

[28] Reuben A. Kessel, "Price Discrimination in Medicine," *Journal of Law and Economics*, vol. 1 (1958).

[29] No one seems to have suggested making blood donors legally responsible for the quality of their blood. Why not?

to develop new skills for discriminating among blood donors in which they have no comparative advantage. The profession opposes it because, although for the majority the lowest-cost blood of given quality is preferred since it is a complementary input to other monopolized professional services, a small faction within the profession is organized as a pressure group. This group comprises those doctors employed in the allegedly more doctor-intensive sector of the blood-supply industry—according to Kessel, the voluntary-donor sector—who have an employment interest at stake.

The Coase theorem implies that, in a world of zero transactions costs, the assignment of liability is irrelevant to the efficiency of outcomes so long as liability is assigned to someone.[30] Kessel argues that, in the case of blood, the assignment of liability *does* matter for efficiency because of asymmetry in the information available to doctors, patients, hospitals, and blood banks. In general, only the doctor is in a position to assess efficiently the information available about a patient and the quality of blood with which he may be transfused. While the other agents may be able to obtain this information, they could do so only at relatively high costs. These costs could be avoided by assigning liability to the physician.

While Kessel's asymmetry argument seems to make a lot of sense, his preceding *explanatory* analysis of the suppliers' and profession's opposition to suppliers' liability seems to make much less sense. If blood banks do not have a comparative advantage in screening out bad blood, it is hard to imagine who has. There is, after all, no shortage of textbooks for blood banks, some of which have been written by their employees.[31] Similarly, I find it hard to believe—at least without more direct evidence—that the American Medical Association's attitude is determined by a small but well-organized minority whose principal interest is to preserve their own jobs. It seems more plausible to argue that the AMA would oppose professional liability because this would reduce professional incomes. With asymmetrical information, the increase in fees that would go along with physician liability would cause a greater fall in income than would the increase in the price of blood since the demand for blood is probably rather price-inelastic, especially if patients are insured. Moreover, with asymmetry in information, law suits for malpractice bring unfavorable publicity to which doctors may be more vulnerable than other suppliers. Alternatively, one could argue that the profession *opposes* liability because it *supports* full voluntarism on the grounds either that patients should have the best quality blood regardless of cost and that voluntarism provides both cheaper *and* better blood anyway. The medical profession, of course,

---

[30] Ronald H. Coase, "The Problem of Social Cost," *Journal of Law and Economics*, vol. 3 (1960).

[31] For example, D. W. Huestis, J. R. Bove, and S. Busch, *Practical Blood Transfusion* (Boston: Little, Brown and Company, 1969).

is famous among economists for its devotion, at least in principle, to "the best regardless of cost." And we are also surely aware that Titmuss's writings have had immense influence despite the fact that they fail crucially to provide either theory or fact to convince us that commercialism in blood collection cannot, suitably designed, produce more blood of any desired quality. Moreover, even if it were the case that the efficient outcome is independent of the initial assignment of liability, individuals are plainly not indifferent to the wealth distributional consequences of such assignments, and wealth, unlike efficient allocations, is not determined only at the margin. A final qualification is that the Coase theorem's prediction that resource allocation is invariate with respect to the initial assignment of liability is also valid only for profit-maximizing parties. With utility-maximizing parties, different initial assignments have different "income" or "welfare" effects which can lead to different—even though efficient—outcomes of exchange.

To toss another pebble into the water, liability seems to me most appropriately fixed on the collection agencies on the joint grounds that they are in the best position to obtain the highest-quality blood—*using whatever techniques they find most effective to that end*—and that the available evidence seems to suggest that the additional costs of collecting blood of very high quality are almost certain to be less than the costs of the consequences of hepatitis.[32]

The argument thus returns to the mainly factual questions that concerned us at the beginning and to the quality of the evidence that bears upon them.

Fraundorf has recently argued that a perfectly competitive blood-banking industry would produce optimality but that the absence of two necessary conditions for effective competition prevents this. These are profit maximization[33] and adequate consumer knowledge of blood quality; the latter, he asserts, requires nonmarket intervention "to do what adequately informed consumers would do themselves, that is, reject diseased blood."[34]

The absence of profit motivation is not, of course, a sufficient condition for inefficiency. As Solow rightly said in rebuking Cooper and Culyer for an overstatement: ". . . it is certainly gratuitous to assert that doctors and hospital administrators respond, presumably necessarily respond, to *no other* stimulus but money. That assertion is not itself economics: it is psychology, and very likely bad psychology."[35] The slip is a common one, but no less excusable for that. Johnson for example wrote: "most hospitals are non-competitive and not profit-

---

[32] Kessel, "Transfused Blood, Serum Hepatitis, and the Coase Theorem," p. 270, estimated the value, in terms of costs avoided of an expected hepatitis case, to be $156 per bottle of blood.

[33] Using data from the National Heart and Lung Institute, 1972, Fraundorf estimates that only 11.2 percent of collections are made by profit organizations.

[34] Kenneth C. Fraundorf, "Competition in Blood Banking," *Public Interest*, vol. 23 (1975), p. 222.

[35] Solow, "Blood and Thunder," p. 1706.

oriented, and thus do not have the incentive to economise."[36] The truth, of course, is that they will—like everyone else—economize but they will economize on different entities from competitive, profit-oriented firms. Where the capital and product markets are such as to permit the survival of nonprofit institutions, it is commonplace to predict utility-maximizing behavior by the management of these institutions. Since it is perfectly possible for there to be limited congruence between the objectives of such managements and the objectives of society, the possibility of inefficiency from the "social" perspective arises. It is, of course, in the context of utility-maximizing behavior by government agencies that some see cost-benefit analysis as a behavior-shaping practice.[37] Not surprisingly, therefore, we find that the blood-collecting industry in the United States is divided by profound differences over objectives and methods. The Red Cross, which collects approximately one-half of the U.S. blood supply, bitterly opposes any form of commercialism in blood transactions: it collects its blood supply from volunteers and charges the hospitals only a processing fee. The hospital and community blood banks, on the other hand, typically use replacement fees in addition to processing fees whereby transfused patients may have their replacement fees returned if they or their friends or relatives replace blood. They also, at least partially, rely on paid donors.[38] The prices charged to hospitals and patients and paid to donors vary enormously by blood product, region, and institution, while philosophical differences add to the difficulty of coordination. In such an institutional setting it seems to add little to one's insight to "explain" the philosophical differences in terms of the pecuniary advantages to the decision makers as Kessel does—just as it would be gratuitously insulting (and plain wrong) to suppose that Titmuss's advocacy of pure voluntarism was motivated by pecuniary considerations.

Fraundorf's surprising solution to these difficulties (after twenty pages discussing competition) is to recommend as a kind of *deus ex machina* the complete monopolization of blood collection by a nonprofit organization such as the Red Cross. Unfortunately, he offers no reasons why we should expect nonprofit monopoly to perform better than nonprofit competition. He offers no conjectures about the size of total supply as unpaid blood replaces paid, about prices to be charged to hospitals, about the quality of blood such a system would produce compared with alternative systems, or about the total cost of such a move.

Much of the literature concerning the blood industry simply assumes that the grass is greener on the other side of the fence. The deficiencies of one system are fallaciously supposed to constitute a sufficient reason for preferring some other system. There is no shortage of theories, but there is precious little *relevant*

---

[36] David B. Johnson, "The U.S. Market in Blood," in Alchian et al., *Economics of Charity*, p. 163.

[37] For example, Roland N. McKean, "Property Rights within Government, and Devices to Increase Governmental Efficiency," *Southern Economic Journal*, vol. 39 (1972).

[38] Titmuss, *Gift Relationship*, p. 93.

evidence enabling one to form a set of reasoned expectations about the consequences of alternative institutional forms. Even the more sympathetic reviewers of Titmuss's book doubt his diagnosis of the causes of some, if not all, the phenomena found in the U.S. blood market.[39]

Evaluating the Evidence

A word of caution is perhaps appropriate concerning evidence. Titmuss has been much criticized for the way he handled his empirical material, and—while, in my view, much of this criticism was justified—the question remains as to what evidence is persuasive. In defending Titmuss against Arrow, Singer argued:

> The extent to which it is reasonable to demand conclusive or very strong evidence before a proposition is taken seriously must vary with the nature of the proposition that is being considered. In a case like the comparison of blood supply systems in different countries, where controlled experiments are impossible and the factor under examination can never be isolated from other differences between the systems, it is unreasonable to demand conclusive proof or anything near it. *Some* genuine evidence there must of course be, before we accept, even tentatively, the view that a commercial system discourages altruism; but once there is some evidence, the onus is on whoever denies this to produce counter-evidence.[40]

How then might one evaluate the evidence concerning the effects of commercialism on the supply of blood and the quality of that supply? My suggestions are listed below.

Relevant Empirical Issues. In the United States an increase in paid donations has been accompanied, it would seem, by a decrease in unpaid donations. If this is a "fact," does it imply that, at some price, total supplies (allowing for the complete withdrawal of unpaid donors and the switching of some of these to the paid section) cannot be made as large as one wishes? Clearly the evidence has no relevance at all to the question of supply elasticity. The only evidence on this point with which I am acquainted comes from a small survey by Ireland and Koch, who found a supply curve with a negative slope at low prices and a positive slope, with elasticity approaching zero, at very high prices. At prices around fifty dollars per unit, however, the "hypothetical" supply was three times larger than that at zero price.[41] Granted this evidence is not very good, what is the counter-evidence?

---

[39] For example, Nathan Glazer, "Blood," *Public Interest*, vol. 24 (1971).

[40] P. Singer, "Altruism and Commerce: A Defense of Titmuss against Arrow," *Philosophy and Public Affairs*, vol. 2 (1973), p. 314.

[41] Ireland and Koch, "Blood and American Social Attitudes."

In the United States more blood is "wasted," in the Titmuss sense, than in Britain. If this is a "fact," is it attributable to paying donors? The hypothesis attributing it to paying donors is not refuted by the evidence that in Seattle (which uses overwhelmingly nonpaid blood) "waste" is but 2 percent compared with New York's 15 percent. But there is another tenable hypothesis: namely, that in the Seattle area a single centralized system monitors local demand and supply closely, while New York has no such coordination. Decentralization with attenuation of profit seeking is thus a hypothesis equally supported by the "facts" as the hypothesis of "rampant commercialism." So the facts do not speak for themselves and Singer's brusque dismissal of Arrow's plea for theory from Titmuss cannot be accepted: there *is* a need for hypotheses whose implications are different and testable and for evidence which would enable us to discriminate between them.

Setting aside questions of quality, the cost of bought blood is higher than that of donated blood. The principal question here relates to marginal opportunity costs. In an efficient system the marginal cost of blood from paid sources should be set at a level equal to that of blood from unpaid sources. We know neither the current relative opportunity costs nor, a fortiori, have we much idea of what they will be in the future. It may be that, at the margin, unpaid blood is less costly. If so, the relative expansion of that sector would be efficient. No one, however, has presented any evidence *at all* on relative marginal costs.

There can be no doubt whatsoever that commercial blood drawn from current sources carries a higher risk than blood from unpaid donors. But this is not evidence for the view that paid blood from more carefully chosen sources would be more risky than unpaid blood. There is a theoretical reason for expecting paid blood from individuals with particular characteristics (for example, nonprisoners, nonaddicts) to be riskier than unpaid since payment provides an incentive to lie. This hypothesis has not, however, been tested empirically. There is, moreover, a counterhypothesis: that what motivates some unpaid donors is the desire *to be seen* doing good deeds, and this also provides an incentive to lie. The fact that blood donors receive certificates and often sport badges suggests that they are not indifferent to public recognition. The validity or relative strength of these effects is an empirical issue about which there is no evidence. Titmuss's questionnaire technique was, of course, unlikely to produce evidence of somewhat "unworthy" motives.

What Can We Infer? On almost any reasonable criterion we may concede that the American system of blood collection is less efficient than the British. Does it follow either that the British system cannot be improved or that Americans ought to copy, so far as possible, British institutions? Manifestly the evidence does not support either inference. There is no more *factual* basis for supposing that granting the American Red Cross a monopoly of blood collection in the United States would produce adequate supplies at the right times with minimal disease-risk than there is for supposing that a profit-seeking collecting industry with strict liability for supplying hazardous blood and, of course, freedom to collect blood by whatever means it found expedient would do the same. Nor is there any compelling *factual* evidence to suggest that stricter regulation and coordination of existing collecting agencies is preferable to either of the foregoing. An assessment of the evidence is not made easier by the welter of merely descriptive and/or completely irrelevant or manifestly false "facts" that have sometimes been adduced in this debate, such as the statement that payments for blood "inflate" the GNP or that they constitute a regressive transfer from the poor to the rich. Most of us have, in the course of this debate, been guilty of occasional overstatement, un-critical acceptance of evidence, and careless injection of implicit values. My own judgment, which I make as impartially as I can, is that to date we have made considerable advances in our theoretical understanding of the blood industry but that we still lack the relevant empirical evidence even to reach a tentative conclusion about the five empirical issues outlined above. Clearly, the argument is not at an end, though we may hope that it will in future include fewer ideologues and theorists and a higher proportion of good empiricists able to tackle those empirical questions to which "reasonably conclusive" answers are, prima facie, attainable.

The Grander Thesis. Interwoven with Titmuss's arguments about blood was a larger and grander theme for which the blood-donation issue was but an illustration. The issues raised by this more fundamental discussion are extremely interesting as well as important for social policy and the whole flavor of society.

In a nutshell, Titmuss's book was a paean for altruism and his arguments on the subject of blood, interpreted in this wider context, were designed to show that the cash nexus of the market destroys altruism, neighborliness, and so on. Since I have little to add to what I have written elsewhere on the issues involved here[42] and am poorly acquainted with the Marxian literature on alienation, I shall make only a few observations whose purpose is no more than to indicate that there is much more of both analytical and ethical interest than Titmuss chose to write about.

It is useful to distinguish *altruism*, defined as a state of mind or an individual's *attitude* towards others, from *generosity*, defined as *behavior* in which resources are voluntarily transferred at less than the maximum economic gain to their initial owner. If this distinction is tenable, several implications follow for the present debate. Some are of particular interest.

(1) Since generosity is observable behavior, we may hypothesize that it is affected by variables commonly considered by economists to affect behavior.

---

[42] Anthony J. Culyer, "*Quids* without *Quos*—A Praxeological Approach," in Alchian et al., *Economics of Charity*.

In particular, generous persons may not actually be altruists and genuine altruists may not be very generous. It follows that the measured degree of generosity in a society is not a reliable indicator of the degree of altruism.

(2) Since altruism describes aspects of a person's utility function, particularly those aspects concerning how he values other people's welfare, and generosity describes his behavior when he maximizes a (possibly nonaltruistic) utility function subject to changing constraints, there is no reason to follow Arrow in supposing that there is a fixed "stock" of altruism to be "used up."[43]

(3) If payment for blood replaces or supplements unpaid donation, there is no reason (subject to considerations under point [4] below) to suppose that those who cease supplying altogether become less altruistic or that those who become paid donors become less altruistic. The former will have become less generous with their blood and the latter may become more or less generous with their blood.[44]

(4) We know remarkably little about the formation of preferences in general and about the fostering of altruism in particular. Singer cites some evidence from Wright showing that *generous* acts tend to promote, *ceteris paribus*, further generous acts by those witnessing them; hence, by example generous acts promote *altruism* since the only explanation for the change in the witnesses's behavior is a change in his attitude, which has presumably become more altruistic.[45]

Now what if it *is* true that in the long—perhaps not so long—run altruism requires the example of generosity, even if generosity of the purest sort (without any cash nexus), to nourish and sustain it?

This, it would seem, is the true heart of the matter. Titmuss drew our attention to it, and the question is still with us despite the fact that it is often put in a rather smug and self-righteous way.[46] The issue will become particularly sharp if "the facts" eventually reveal that paying donors is actually a more effective way of meeting the clinical needs of modern medicine than soliciting

---

[43] Arrow, "Gifts and Exchanges," p. 335.

[44] See also David B. Johnson, "The Charity Market Theory and Practice," in Alchian et al., *Economics of Charity*, pp. 88-89.

[45] D. Wright, *The Psychology of Moral Behavior* (London: Penguin Books, 1971).

[46] For example, A. Kliman in "Gold vs. The Gift of Blood," *New England Journal of Medicine*, vol. 287 (1972) writes: "Paying students to donate blood is especially repugnant since it is in fact the responsibility of the medical profession to teach young people not to sell blood but to give blood willingly for humanitarian reasons without demanding payment." (p. 51) Kliman does not assert that it is the responsibility of physicians to give their services willingly for humanitarian reasons without demanding payment. It is not actually a "fact" that the profession bears this responsibility. But it is a "fact" that Kliman is implicitly drawing on some ethical principles concerning the "responsibility" or "duty" of citizens toward one another. By failing to make it explicit he begs the whole crucial question that concerns us in the present context.

donations, for then the mysticism that seems inherent in Titmuss's view will clash directly with the utilitarian consequences of that same view; the assertion of the absolute value of the gift as an end in itself will confront the assertion of its pragmatic and instrumental role as a means to another worthy end.[47]

My own tentative judgment is that the blood market issues are best resolved on their own merits; it is hard to see them, except for illustrative purposes, as anything other than peripheral to the grander issue of the unifying social role of altruism and its central place in the good society. On this wider issue we must be wary of mere sentimentality. Historically, altruism and the love of man have never served as a sufficient foundation for the organization of society. This was and is true of the primitive societies discussed by Titmuss; it is true even of closed and protected Christian communities whose principles include total commitment to the love of God and of man—but whose societies are invariably regulated by rigid authority. Even the liberal order upon which we pride ourselves in the West is a luxury that societies wishing to survive have been able to afford only in modern times.

A not altogether prejudiced interpretation of the values of our own societies would, I think, reveal that the role of altruism is normally regarded as limited: limited, that is, mainly to the most personal of relationships (where it is usually called "love") and to charity, helping those seen to be in "need." I am not aware of compelling evidence that either of these two broad types of altruism is much on the wane in the "civilized" West. Indeed, the rapid extension of social welfare programs in recent decades suggests that the latter type, at least, is on the increase. Self-reliance; mutual respect; friendliness and companionship; pursuit of excellence; careers open to talent; responsibility for one's dependents; competence and reliability at one's job and due recognition of these virtues; the removal of boredom and triviality from the workplace; the pursuit of comfort, beauty, and health; the satisfaction of curiosity; the protection of oneself and one's nearest and dearest from the assaults of nature—these ends, for which the pursuit of wealth is sometimes a necessary means, seem to me to describe, perhaps incompletely, yet more accurately than "altruism," the aspirations of our society and, moreover, to identify a set of shared beliefs. They do not appear to be unethical aspirations or beliefs. And if, in general, there is a case for the market, duly regulated, monitored, and even supplemented, as the most appropriate *general* mechanism yet devised by man for their attainment, then the market—together with accountable, "democratic," but inevitably coercive, government—cannot be dismissed as an unethical "commercial" instrument for promoting them.

---

[47] It is not made absolutely clear in Titmuss's discussion whether the gift relationship itself is really best seen as instrumental. Certainly, in the case of blood he regards it as a more efficient *means* than commercial exchange. As a *general* proposition, however, the gift viewed solely as a means of efficient allocation would surely not bear much scrutinizing and Titmuss himself avers: "That [altruism] may, incidentally, create economic wealth by sustaining life is subsidiary in conception, conduct and objective." *Gift Relationship*, p. 212.

In short, the *general* case for altruism either as an end or as a means remains to be made. While it would be unreasonable to place a heavy burden of proof on those who assert the contrary, I (along, I suspect, with most of my fellow creatures) will need more evidence and a fuller theoretical explanation before I can even ascribe plausibility to the case for the overriding social value of the gift relationship.

To end on a speculative note: I hazard that the impact of Titmuss's book, which has been remarkable, is largely attributable to what Arrow describes as its

> resonant evocation of central problems of social value. His blithe disregard of the usual epistemological structures against confusion of act and value permits him to raise the largest descriptive and normative questions about the social order in a highly specific and highly factual context. . . . By suggestively combining a passionately informed commitment to an ideal social order and an illustration of problems within the context of a concrete situation, it has greatly enriched the quality of social-philosophical debate.[48]

Its success is largely due to its rejection of positivism, whose victory has otherwise been all too complete, especially in economics. There is a lesson here for us all— not that we should follow Titmuss in methodological error but that we should be far less casual than we commonly are in our value judgments; far less "loaded" in our positivistic applications of theory and, when occasion demands, passionate in our explication of the relationships between economic processes and institutions on the one hand and conceptions of the ideal social order on the other. What was good for Frank Knight cannot be too bad for the rest of us. If positivism has taught us to keep prediction and prescription apart (or at least remote), which is useful, Titmuss has taught us to respect the impact of commitment and advocacy. Reason, I believe, teaches us that neither is enough.

---

[48] Arrow, "Gifts and Exchanges," p. 362.

COMMENTARIES

Mike Reddin

I want to begin with a brief restatement of some lines from Titmuss about the relevance of the British experience for the United States. Towards the end of *The Gift Relationship* Titmuss wrote:

> The assumption should not be drawn from the comparative material presented in this study that, in terms of moral values, there is anything particularly unique or meritorious about the British people in their commitment to and support of a voluntary blood donor programme. In many other countries besides Britain and the United States, there are doubtless numbers of voluntary community donors. If asked, there is no reason to doubt that many would respond by expressing similar sentiments of altruism and reciprocity. . . . But just because we have presented a mass of facts about voluntary donors in Britain and few facts about volunteers in other countries, there must not, we repeat, be thoughts about chosen people.[1]

Developments in Britain and the United States

I want to refer briefly to developments in the United Kingdom since 1967 and 1968 (the last years for which Richard Titmuss studied substantial data) and review some similar developments in the United States. I want to comment specifically, if briefly, on points raised in two of today's contributions—Clark Havighurst's paper which I heard this morning and Tony Culyer's paper which he sent me some weeks ago. Finally, I want to reexamine the characteristics of the U.S. donor and express my concern for the future development of blood policy.

Since 1968 there have been few dramatic developments in the National Blood Transfusion Service in the United Kingdom; its pattern of organization has remained broadly unchanged within the recently reorganized National Health Service, a pattern of relatively autonomous regional services with extensive co-operation between regions. Both the number of donors and the number of donations have steadily grown.

Since Titmuss wrote, apart from continuing technological developments which are generally comparable to those taking place in the United States, some small

---

[1] Richard M. Titmuss, *The Gift Relationship* (London: Allen and Unwin, 1970), pp. 224-25.

changes have occurred in the use of plasmapheresis by the National Blood Transfusion Service. Each region is free to conduct plasmapheresis and some now choose to do so. For example, one of the southern London regions has a plasmapheresis program in which about 700 volunteers currently participate about once a week, almost all of them female, almost all married. (I will consider the significance of this donor group later.)

Since 1968 donations have grown in the United Kingdom by some 25 percent. For comparison, let me draw attention to the fact (not mentioned in this debate) that over the same period the American Red Cross (ARC) has experienced an increase of donations of 46 percent, a rise from some 2.9 million donations in 1967 to 4.2 million in 1974–1975. If we extrapolate from the figures for the first nine months, the ARC will collect in excess of 4.5 million units of blood this year (a quantity which still, I believe, understates the ARC potential). Most of the technological changes that have taken place in Britain, as in the United States, are related to the increased use of blood components. Research continues to be much concerned with improving techniques for identifying impure blood and for "washing" or purifying it. Some of the research in Britain is being conducted jointly with institutions in this country, and there is considerable interchange of research ideas and information, particularly through the respective national agencies involved in this field.

Reservations about Legal Solutions

Let me comment briefly on points raised in Professor Havighurst's paper and then in that of Tony Culyer before looking again at U.S. donors and donor systems.

If I may use his own phrase, I take Professor Havighurst to be a moderately well-born American. Nonetheless, I think both he and Professor Kessel overstate the self-interest and bad intentions of medical professionals while apparently denying the professional self-interest of lawyers. Their solution—continuing to use the courts to blast hepatitis off the face of the earth—seems to me rather like enrolling the National Rifle Association to eliminate street violence in America.

The law lacks subtlety. Even in the specific examples, relating court action to subsequent blood use, much of the response one sees may be the reaction to labeling procedures per se—and not simply the result of tort liability. I do not deny that laws have impact; I merely question the impact of specific laws in specific situations in the United States today. I find little to convince me of the beneficent contributions that the law has made to the practice of medicine and to health care in the United States—particularly when I observe other developed societies which have improved their care without lawyers' obsessively following each flick of the knife and drip of the transfusion. How on earth do the rest of us survive without the legal attentions Havighurst and Kessel insist we need?

In passing, I must express my concern about some of the sentiments implicit and explicit at the start of Clark Havighurst's paper—for instance, the imputations of sinister motive and bias in Titmuss's work. The suggestion that as a Socialist he is necessarily prejudiced seems to me an unwarranted juxtaposition, just as the association of the prefix *capitalist* with the term *lawyer* should not, of itself, be presumed to remove from the lawyer in question any possibility of intelligent thought. I would be happier if we could set aside the question of motives—unless we were to examine the motives of all of the contributors to this conference. I promise not to mention the matter further!

Broad Social Issues

Let me now pursue a couple of issues raised in Tony Culyer's paper, although they merit much more attention than these precious minutes allow. I agree with most of his analysis, but must, of necessity, concentrate on the points where I disagree.

Partly my objections hinge on the fact that Culyer, Havighurst, and other contributors focus too narrowly on blood. If we concentrate so exclusively on "maximum efficiencies," on "states of optimality" in the blood market, we can either incur complementary social costs that we might wish to avoid or negate other social objectives that we might wish to pursue. Culyer does not ignore, but seems to minimize, this danger.

My interest focuses on the point where societies make large-scale general decisions; where they express the wish to move in a "macro" direction which might well not be compatible with optimally efficient decisions at the "micro" level. For example, a general wish to pursue social policies that integrate rather than segregate citizens might be incompatible with the optimality of some smaller-scale objective, such as the recruitment of blood donors in the simplest, cheapest, most efficient way available. I would prefer to see the latter issue resolved in the light of the larger objective; I am uncertain how this resolution is aided by tort liabilities, but I acknowledge that economists can at least illuminate the apparent incompatibilities of micro optimalities within macro world views!

In his paper Culyer comments on his earlier failure to discuss the problem of serum hepatitis. My own thoughts, with hindsight, are that it was no bad thing to leave that issue out of the broader debate about blood donation, recruitment policies, and so on. There is great danger in a purely pragmatic response to the issue of hepatitis and its identification. If someone were to solve this problem tomorrow he would not, to my mind, resolve the dilemmas of donor recruitment. There are those involved in the debate on hepatitis detection who secretly wish that solutions, rather like cures for VD, would never be discovered so that certain "moral" restraints in the fight against the commercial donor would remain in force. We are probably close to being able to identify the hepatitis carrier. When we can, will a large segment of the National Blood Policy fall apart?

I think it crucial that the argument about the future role of voluntary or nonvoluntary blood donation in society should not hinge on this technical breakthrough. I am very concerned about who is going to be allowed to donate in our societies and on what terms. The task of social scientists, Culyer comments, is not to identify the proper arbiters of blood-collection policy; I would add that it can and should be part of the social scientist's task to consider the consequences of choosing one set of arbiters (and their chosen set of arbitrating mechanisms) rather than another.

Let me offer a practical illustration. If we want to enable as many people as possible to give, we must support inclusive rather than exclusive screening programs for blood donors. The evidence of serum hepatitis among U.S. donors points to a correlation between a socioeconomic variable and infected blood, in the past most conspicuous when money changed hands. The critical policy issue remains whether we wish to encourage all citizens in our society to give blood. If we presume this to have some useful social connotations (and I deliberately say *if*) then our recruitment programs and our research policy must flow from that decision. If we are not interested in who gives blood as long as we receive the amount and the quality we want, then we pursue some mix of the policies that have been followed up to now in the United States. Perhaps only another round of litigation and technology stands between us and our quantity and quality targets. If we are actively concerned that the whole range of people in this society should have an opportunity to give blood, then we need to do the following things—and forgive me for being prescriptive.

First, we must seriously examine the impact of the whole credit/contractual approach to blood donation. This strikes me as one of the most glaringly restrictive practices one could devise. The technique of encouraging people to give through clubs or churches, or their families, is likely to produce the first "contractual" donation and to discourage any donations beyond those specifically demanded in the contract. Further, the current Red Cross Family Plan is in effect saying that when one person gives there will be up to eleven or twelve covered relations who therefore need not give. There is no hard American research evidence on this subject (although it would seem easy enough to derive it from existing data held by collection agencies); but in the United Kingdom, where the contractual approach is not used, the families of donors have been one of the strongest and stablest sources of donor recruitment.

The second major characteristic of the U.S. donor population is its maleness; about three out of four donations come from males. Given the fact that the incidence of the hepatitis antigen is two to three times lower in the female population than it is among males, it is crazy to waste all those women. This I associate with the essential "maleness" of the credit/contractual approach; the male is the "good father," the breadwinner, and the blood donor, providing cover for his dependents. If we break the contractual approach we will be in a much stronger position to tap the female potential. With my general concern for a broadbased donor population, I believe this to be crucial.

Nevertheless, I appreciate the problems of breaking the contractual bond in the American blood market. This is a fee-for-service, insurance-laden medical-care delivery system. Even in the nonprofit sector handling charges are involved which donors may well see as being a surcharge on their gift, but I see the major block to gift giving as the profit-making intermediary.

In analyses of the British blood donor system, surprisingly little emphasis has been given to the significance of having a socially approved nonprofit agency (the National Health Service) act as intermediary between donor and recipient, an agency that visibly does *not* profit as it handles, efficiently, the donor's gift. The American donor sees his blood pass through the hands of agencies ranging from the Red Cross to proprietary hospitals, and sees recipients billed via agencies and procedures where the association of handling charges, mark-ups, or simple profit is hard to disentangle.[2] It is this barrier which the American donor has to leap, at the very least psychologically, to break out of the world of contract and restrictive covenant.

I appreciate, of course, that this proposal begs numerous questions about the effects of commercialism on the supply of blood and the interaction of "commercial" and "altruistic" sources. Culyer is right about the shortage of known facts in the area. On the other hand, American researchers have the advantage of observing a society in which a variety of delivery systems are in use. The overlap between these systems might help track down these interrelationships.

Are there indeed clusters of "givers" in our respective societies? Can we observe consistent patterns of human behavior when we look at the extent to which people who give, say, dollars also give blood? Are we, in other words, using up a stock of altruism when people give, or are we encouraging and stimulating it to further growth? Perhaps this is something Professor Drake is going to deal with in reporting on his work this afternoon.

Most of the evidence suggests—including two recent British studies on donors—that motivations are very low-key, very low in "mystery content." Simple convenience—how easily people can get to places to give blood—is a major determinant of much blood donation in the United Kingdom.

One final point. Can we begin to account for the degree of hostility that the

---

[2] The blood coverage practices of American insurance companies vary widely. Some policies cover the processing and replacement costs of blood; others exclude from any coverage the first few units transfused; others pay only for the processing fees and not for the blood replacement fees. Apparently, even the government health programs of Medicare and Medicaid vary in their coverage of blood costs. Where the private insurance company policies do include blood costs, the costs are passed on to the consumer in the form of higher premiums.

proposal for an all-volunteer blood program has generated in the United States? The proposal has produced such delightful documents in recent months as the critique from the Council on Wage and Price Stability.[3] Its authors obviously conceive their response as one further battle for the survival of free enterprise, democracy and the best of bicentennial values, with the ARC as the antichrist and HEW as, presumably, the seven-headed beast. I concede that, by adopting an all-volunteer program, we could be reverting to the values of mutual aid that were espoused in the United States when all-volunteer programs were run in World War II, during the Korean War, and so on. Such apparent neglect of market values may seem subversive to the council even though mutual aid may have a hard time reasserting itself in a contract-pervaded society. Indeed, once such values reemerge, they can open up wider possibilities than the simple gift of blood to strangers. Perhaps it is this confusing prospect of a giving rather than a trading society which causes the council such concern.

Simon Rottenberg

It is possible to define the objectives to be served by a blood-collection and distribution system. Those objectives are:

(1) the collection of optimal quantities of blood of different types;

(2) the optimal distribution of blood stocks in time and space;

(3) the collection of the optimal quality of blood in the blood stock;

(4) the optimal reduction of the quantity of blood that is discarded; and

(5) the achievement of those four objectives at the lowest possible cost in real resources employed in collecting and distributing tasks.

The primary question in the design of blood policy is: What are the properties of a system of collecting and distributing and what are the rules instructing behavior that will best help meet those objectives?

Some clarifying points need to be made about the five objectives. First, optimizing with respect to the quality of blood does not mean reducing to zero the probability that blood transfusion will generate serum hepatitis. High quality in blood, as in other products, is costly. Real resources employed in the production of quality in blood have alternative valuable uses for society, and society forgoes those uses if, in fact, they are put to the task of improving quality in

---

[3] U.S., Congress, House, Filing before the Food and Drug Administration on blood labelling, *Whole Blood and Red Blood Cells*, Docket No. 75N-0316; comments of the Council on Wage and Price Stability, January 13, 1976.

blood. The parameters are likely to be such that it would be too costly and not socially worthwhile to reduce the probability of transmission of hepatitis to zero.

Second, discarded blood is not necessarily wasteful. Titmuss found that more blood was discarded in this country, where some blood is commercially produced and commercially exchanged, than in Britain, and he inferred that there is more waste of blood in this country than in Britain. His inference may have been wrong. Discarding blood does not necessarily imply waste.

Blood banks, hospitals, and surgeons in operating rooms apply inventory strategies. Their work is characterized by uncertainty. They do not know *ex ante* with perfect assurance how much blood of different types they will find it appropriate to use. One way for them to diminish the risk that they will not have blood when it is required is to carry an inventory of blood. The larger the stock, the smaller the risk. But the larger the stock, the higher the probability that some of the blood will outlive its shelf life and will be discarded.

Discarded blood, thus, is a consequence of strategies for diminishing risk, and these are not prima facie bad social policy. There are, of course, such things as suboptimal inventory strategies, excessive storage, excessively diminished risk, and excessive discarding of blood. But the observation that more blood is discarded here than in the United Kingdom does not tell us that medical practice is more wasteful here; it might be more wasteful there, where suboptimal inventory strategies increase the risk that blood will be unavailable when and where it is needed.

Third, real resources are employed in collecting and distributing blood whatever the systemic arrangements. It does not matter whether donors give or sell and whether recipients receive at zero or positive prices. In all cases— altruistic and commercial—resources are consumed in the performance of blood-system tasks. One of the efficiency tests for the ordering of different collection and distribution systems would be their comparative resource costs. It is apparently not known, however, whether the effort and time given to the recruitment of non-commercial donors is larger or smaller, per 1,000 units procured, than that given to the recruitment of commercial donors. Ignorance on this point might well lead to the design of inappropriate blood policy.

Liability, Efficiency, and Tolerable Risk

I pass now to the discussion of the liability rule that will tend to achieve the efficiency objectives defined above. The transfusion of blood will generate serum hepatitis as an adverse side effect with some positive probability. If the adverse effect occurs, damage is done to the patient. The law assigns the duty to repair damage by enforcing some form of a liability role. There are, in principle, three forms of such a rule: (1) there might be strict liability, as when the law compels the provider—physician, blood bank, or hospital—to repair or compensate for the damage upon the simple evidence that hepatitis was contracted and without examining whether the provider was negligent; (2) there might be fault liability, which would compel the provider to repair damage if, and only if, he were negligent in the sense of exercising less caution than the standard of prudent practice of his community required of him; or (3) there might be zero liability lodged upon the provider, and the patient might assume the risk (and bear the cost of repair) of contracting hepatitis after the transfusion of blood. In the zero provider-liability case, the provider might warrant only that he delivered blood derived from sources having prescribed characteristics, but he would not warrant purity and would not be held liable if hepatitis ensued.

Which of these rules would tend to optimize caution in collecting blood? Accepted community practice with respect to other products and other aspects of behavior may be instructive. We find it acceptable to permit people to run risks. We do not require that purchasers of automobiles buy only those with roll bars installed so that the roof will not crush them if the car should roll over. We do not prevent them from buying unbranded drugs bearing only generic names, with unknown qualities of bio-availability (that is, the capacity of the human body to assimilate the therapeutic effects of a drug). So, with a host of products, we permit transaction of both high- and low-quality models, types, and brands. We permit the sale and purchase of models with which there are associated both high and low probabilities of the occurrence of adverse side effects. Similarly, we find it tolerable to permit risky occupational tasks to be done and risky recreational ventures to be undertaken. We do not foreclose the painting of steeples and the washing of high windows, even though they may produce broken backs; we do not foreclose the underground mining of coal, though it may produce black lung disease or death from explosions or entrapment by fallen stone. We permit the climbing of mountains and the running of rapids.

Safety is costly. Products with guards over moving parts cost more than those without guards. Drugs with side effects that are kept off the market are forestalled from use as therapeutic instruments to meliorate pain and cure disease. If coal were not mined home heating and power-generating resources would be more scarce. In general society confronts the problem of risk by permitting choice to be made within the limits of very broad discretionary authority lodged in individuals. Individuals are confronted by products that are more or less safe and that are offered at higher and lower prices, and they are permitted to choose.

Social policies that permit choice and tolerate risk are attractive on two grounds. First, they are consistent with the existence of freedom of the individual. Second, they tend towards the maximization of the welfare of society. They tend towards welfare-maximization, while a social policy that forecloses to the individual the selection of relatively less safe, less expensive products diminishes the number of alternatives and compels him to buy an increment of safety for some fraction of his income that he might have preferred to spend on some other commodity or service. In the jargon of the economists, such a policy moves the individual along his budget line to a point on a lower indifference curve than that reflecting free choice. A policy proscribing relatively unsafe goods makes the people worse off and compels them to acquire a basket of commodities and services other than those preferred. Since, given their incomes, it is the poor who tend to buy lower-quality commodities, such a policy adversely affects the poor more than the well-to-do. It is regressive in its effects; it transfers income and wealth from the poor to the rich; it makes the poor relatively worse off and the rich relatively better off.

The Implications for Blood Policy

Blood is not different from other commodities with respect to the properties just discussed. Blood can be differentiated in principle as being of high quality or low. Some blood lots have low and some high probabilities of the transmission of hepatitis. Some blood is drawn from members of the Union League Club and deacons of the Episcopal church, and some is drawn from the denizens of skid rows.

The safer blood is made to be, the more costly it is. Cutting off the donations of skid row habitués means that more resources must be devoted to rousing the altruistic enthusiasm and recruiting the gift of some given quantity of blood by deacons of the church. Society loses the valuable output of those resources in alternative uses or it must offer deacons of the church a higher price.

Social welfare would tend to be maximized if recipients were offered an array of blood lots of different qualities at different prices and if they were permitted to choose among them. If individuals are not in a position to choose or if society has organized institutional arrangements that permit providers to act as agents of the recipients in choosing, it is then appropriate to form a set of rules that would tend to make the de facto choosers "honest." By this I mean that the rules ought to instruct them to make the choices that would have been made by the recipients if *they* had, in fact, executed the choice.

It is this principle that gives me pause with respect to the rule placing strict liability upon providers. It is a rule that compels providers to repair damage. It gives them incentives to search for "pure" blood with the lowest possible probability of hepatitic infection. They engage in that search not at their own cost, but rather at the cost of the recipient or of an insurance pool or of the general community. It is a rule that compels the members of the community to secure higher-quality blood than they want, given its cost. It is a rule that produces an excess of caution and diminishes risk to a suboptimal level.

On the other hand, a possible defense for the strict-liability rule may lie in the argument that providers can be cautious at the lowest cost and, therefore, that the rule ought compel *them* to execute the cautionary function. But there are some data on the distribution of medical histories of hepatitis among different subsets of the population from which probabilities of infection can be derived for different blood lots taken from different donor sets. This information, together with price information for lots of different quality, can be given to recipients' kinfolk who can act as surrogates in choosing.

Providers might then be held by the law to warrant the donor class from which the lot was taken. Error might be held in check by the threat of suit for breach of contract and fraud by threat of criminal charge. It is not clear, however, that providers can be cautious at the cheapest cost, and the case for strict liability is, I think, an uneasy one.

I conclude these comments by addressing a central concern of this conference: Are altruistic arrangements for securing blood from donors to be preferred to commercial arrangements?

I conclude that they are not. Like the rule of strict liability, altruistic donor arrangements are intended to shut out blood lots which are characterized by somewhat higher probabilities of communicating hepatitis to recipients. A strategy to foreclose the commercial organization of blood markets might well produce an excess of caution. Altruistic arrangements also sacrifice quantity of donated blood in order to achieve higher blood quality. The trade-off that transpires might well be suboptimal.

Altruistic arrangements offer blood to recipients at a zero price. Zero prices almost invariably result in waste of social resources. They imply an absence of signals to instruct decision makers so that they may be socially productive and will take account of the relative scarcity of resources and the relative degree of need. They also foreclose opportunities for the mutually advantageous and consensual exchanges that occur in commercial markets.

The proposed altruistic arrangements for the blood supply and distribution system are defective as an instrument to achieve higher ethical standards. They encourage impersonal compassion or sharing that lacks moral content because donors and recipients are not known to each other and there is no tenderness or love or caring in the relationship. Tested by standards of both efficiency and ethics, altruistic systems seem not to be superior to commercial systems. It is truly a source of wonder that Professor Titmuss's notions have made so much progress in the blood community.

Arthur N. Levine

Professor Titmuss took the view that, with respect to the blood-supply system, the goal should be to keep risks at a technical minimum. Professor Havighurst has presented the position that various incentives must be considered (he has one in mind in particular) to produce high-quality blood and that there should be a combination of strategies. Finally, Professor Culyer, in his prepared remarks, argued that the risk differential with respect to hepatitis was subject to empirical verification but observed that whether any particular differential was acceptable was a value judgment, which he felt he was not compelled to make. My client, the Food and Drug Administration, is obliged to make judgments of that kind, and I would now like to briefly outline the judgments that the FDA has exercised in order to create "incentives" and minimize risks in the collection and distribution of high-quality blood to the public.

The Position of the FDA

Blood, its components, and its derivatives are drugs within the meaning of the federal Food, Drug and Cosmetic Act and therefore are subject to regulatory authority under that act. Blood, its components, and its derivatives are also biological products within the meaning of the Public Health Service Act and are subject to licensure and regulations standards under that act.

The Food and Drug Act requires, at a minimum, that all drugs which move in interstate commerce must be neither adulterated nor misbranded. A drug is adulterated if it is processed in a manner that does not comply with current good manufacturing practices. A drug is misbranded if its labeling is false or misleading in any particular or if its labeling fails to state a material fact.

The Public Health Service Act provides that all biological drugs must be licensed to move in interstate commerce. To obtain a license, the applicant must present data showing that the product will be safe, pure, and potent, and the licensee must comply with federal regulations. Because blood can transmit a communicable disease, hepatitis, it is subject to additional statutory powers authorizing all appropriate measures, including the promulgation of regulations, to inhibit the spread of such diseases. Finally, under the authority of the Public Health Service Act, too, biological products such as blood and its derivatives and components cannot be labeled in a way that is false or misleading.

Pursuant to this statutory scheme, the Food and Drug Administration has established regulations designed to ensure that blood is of a consistently high quality and that the risk of the transmission of hepatitis is minimized.

There have been four major regulatory actions recently. In November 1975, regulations defining good manufacturing practices for blood banks, transfusion facilities, and plasmapheresis centers were promulgated. These include guidelines for personnel, facilities, and equipment, ancillary supplies and reagents, collection and production controls, laboratory controls, compatability testing, and record keeping.

The Food and Drug Administration has also required licenses and adherence to manufacturing standards for all plasma collected by plasmapheresis. Critical elements of the plasmapheresis regulations include guidelines for donor suitability, limits on the amount a donor can be bled, and definitions of proper medical supervision and informed consent. Similar regulations and licensure have existed for many years with respect to whole blood and red blood cells but only in the last three years has the government licensed plasma derived by plasmapheresis.

The third element is the requirement that each donation of blood, plasma, or serum be tested for hepatitis. Pursuant to regulations published in July 1975, only testing of the third-generation sensitivity is acceptable. Our regulations severely restrict the use of hepatitis-containing blood; donors who are known to be carriers of hepatitis, of course, cannot be bled.

Finally (and I think this will be a subject of discussion this afternoon), the FDA has recently proposed to require that the labeling of blood indicate whether it has been collected from paid or unpaid donors and include a warning that blood collected from paid donors is associated with a higher risk of transmitting hepatitis.

Those are the basic pieces of the regulatory strategy in the government's incentive system. How they compare with the systems discussed by Professor Havighurst is to be determined. There has been a suggestion this morning that there exist economic incentives in the private sector which will regulate blood quality. I have found, regrettably, that there is often an incentive in the private sector to "get by." Government regulations are minimum requirements designed to curtail "getting by" and to create a bottom line.

As to strict and other forms of liability, the Food and Drug Administration can take both prospective and retrospective action—injunctions to prevent the dissemination of adulterated drugs and misbranded drugs, including blood, and the seizure of blood already on the market if it is adulterated or misbranded. The FDA may suspend or revoke blood or plasma product licenses for failure to comply with published standards or the terms of a license. Ultimately, criminal prosecution, which is based upon strict liability and does not require a showing of wrongdoing or intent to commit a crime, may be instituted.

As a lawyer I feel compelled to note the general philosophy discussed in Professor Havighurst's paper, which is that social policy can be determined by private lawyers litigating singular fact situations (malpractice being a current example) and that such suits can establish priorities, economic and otherwise, within an industry. Whether private lawyers or other decision makers, such as the Congress or expert federal agencies, are better qualified to establish such policies and implementing programs is a question that could be debated for the remainder of the afternoon and probably the remainder of the month. It seems to me, however, that the public participatory forum of government is more likely to ensure broad medical and lay contributions to formulating public policy than the often circumscribed presentation of issues in private litigation.

Timm M. Hurst

Apparently I am the only morning discussant actively engaged in blood banking. This places me in the position of representing that nonprofit sector of providers categorized by Clark Havighurst as lacking the incentive to improve upon quality of service and as ill-equipped to select the best solution from among many alternative solutions. Peter Drucker once said of economists, "they have always suffered from one big inherent defect. They love humanity, but they hate human beings." I am beginning to think the same is true of legal academicians.

Definitions

As is the custom in blood banking, it is necessary to comment on the use of certain words to facilitate a common understanding. We have used the word *provider* frequently in conjunction with the identification of legal responsibility. It seems to me that within the blood-service industry there are at least three and possibly four subcategories of providers. One is the attending physician who prescribes the use of blood for patients. Another is the blood bank or blood center charged with the responsibility for selecting the blood donor and collecting and processing the blood. A third is the hospital transfusion service entrusted with the responsibility of ensuring that the donor and recipient blood are compatible. Another provider, more remote, is the supplier of disposables and reagents used in the process. All of these are providers. Each may be a separate legal entity directed by a different board with different motivations and legal responsibilities. It appears to me that this conference is focusing on the responsibility of the blood center.

Commercial is another word in need of further definition. In blood banking it is commonly applied to any organization that pays blood donors. It is also applied to a blood bank incorporated on a for-profit basis. Commercialism is also an attitude or an influence.

Regardless of its specific interpretation, the word *commercialism* generally has a negative connotation in the blood and component market. The sins of some taint the images of all; the commercials are thought of as taking minimum and occasionally substandard precautions in an effort to maximize profits, and for the most part such organizations have contributed minimally to scientific and medical advance in blood. This is principally noteworthy in light of the substantial contributions of many of the nonprofit providers.

Another term worthy of further comment is *the blood market*. I view the blood market as consisting of two submarkets; the link between them is the human being as source and recipient. Between that link are two different channels. One, the blood and component market is characterized by nonprofit blood centers

71

relying primarily on voluntary blood donors. The other, frequently referred to as the plasma market, is a capital-intensive business because of the processing equipment it requires and is dominated by for-profit free-enterprise corporations using cash payments as the primary incentive for donation.

Little attention is being directed to the plasma market today. It should be noted that a major unanswered question in the United States today is, should the policies be the same for both segments of the blood market? The American Enterprise Institute may want to consider this issue in a future seminar.

Incentives, Liability, and Altruism

Now for a few specific comments on today's papers. Dr. Havighurst indicates that the justifications underlying the theory of strict liability are: first, that the provider is in a better position than anyone else to bear the financial burden of the resulting illness; second, that the cost of illness is spread across a broad social base; and third, that strict liability provides the incentive necessary to motivate the health-care provider to improve the quality of care.

On the incentive issue, I would like to say that I personally resent its implications and categorically reject it as a generalization applicable to health care in the United States. Hepatitis will be conquered with or without the lawyers! The incentive to solve this problem came long before the application of strict liability in the *Cunningham* case, and medical research will continue in spite of the potential financial devastation that will hang over many of the scientific investigators engaged in blood banking if strict liability becomes the law of the land.

Another of the implicit supporting theories—the ability to pay—concerns me. The ability to pay whom? What will be the added cost to society in legal bills to prosecute the admittedly increased number of law suits under strict liability? I think Dr. Havighurst, in his paper, probably speaks to this matter better than I can when he says:

> "strict liability in tort" would, if adopted, obviate such proof [of breach of warranty] and would greatly increase not only the frequency of success in prosecuting suits but also the number of suits brought, since lawyers are more likely to accept cases involving low evidence-gathering costs and a high probability of success.

Applying the same logic to the practice of medicine, I feel that I could safely predict a marked reduction in complications resulting from blood transfusions if transfusions were limited to cases where blood was known to be pure and the chances for success were high. We must be thankful that lawyers and doctors go to different schools.

Professor Culyer raises the doubt that altruism is a sufficient incentive to motivate the required number of blood donors in this country. If we could agree on defining *altruism* to mean donation for the benefit of others without a financial reward for the donor or patient, I would offer the following personal experience. Over the past two years my organization—Blood Services—has discontinued the use of cash, replacement credits, insurance, and assurance as donor incentives and has substituted the rationale that people should give their blood because other people need it. The results of this change are encouraging evidence in support of the theory that altruism can work—if the personnel are willing to exert themselves to make it work.

It has been suggested that a free market would cure the problems of the blood market. I find it rather interesting that the incident Havighurst chooses to support this theory comes from Chicago, probably the best example of a city-wide free market in blood practice in this country. It has a Red Cross blood center, approximately six community nonprofit centers, commercial (for-profit) blood centers, and an abundance of hospital-based blood centers. Chicago also has frequent blood shortages, a confused donor public, and an excessively high cost for blood created for the most part by unnecessary duplication of personnel, equipment, and facilities.

On the other hand, there are many examples in this country of excellent community blood programs operating in a quasi-monopolistic environment. Some examples are the programs in Seattle, Portland, San Francisco, Phoenix, Kansas City, Milwaukee, Pittsburgh, Rochester, Atlanta, and Birmingham. One thing they all have in common is a coordinated promotion program that gives a consistent message to the public and a common inventory of blood for all to draw upon. The benefits that Kessel et al. believed could be expected in the blood market through the application of free-enterprise concepts have, in practice, contributed little to the efficiency, quality, or advancement of blood services in this country.

On the positive side, commercialism often conveys the notion of excellence in management and efficiency in performance. Like the hospital industry until a few years ago, blood banks have not attracted the skilled managers so commonplace today in the business world. As a result, many well-established management practices have been slow to be introduced in the blood market. This is gradually changing. It is this form of commercialism or commercial influence that is needed and welcomed by us all.

Irwin Wargon

I have one or two comments on Professor Havighurst's paper. While I take issue with a couple of his minor points, I find myself in agreement with the main thrust of his proposals.

Assignment of Costs and Risks

Professor Havighurst states that strict liability not only would lead to the procurement of safer blood but also would increase the incentives for attending physicians to economize in the utilization of blood supplies. The incentive to greater economy is provided by the indirect assignment of hepatitis risk to attending physicians. The liability, according to Professor Havighurst, would be initially assigned to the hospital and to the blood bank, but low transaction costs would shift an appropriate part of this risk to the attending physician.

Such transactions usually occur among wealth-maximizing parties, but hospitals and blood banks are predominantly nonprofit institutions, while attending physicians are in private practice. When I studied outdating several years ago, I found the following arrangement of property rights between hospitals, blood banks, and pathologists: Blood was collected and distributed to hospitals by the Red Cross. Hospital inventories of blood were controlled by pathologists, the majority of whom operated on "percentage-of-gross" contracts with nonprofit hospitals. Pathologists received a percentage of the cross-match fee for every pint of blood reserved for patients by the attending physicians, regardless whether the blood was actually transfused or returned to inventory. Pathologists, therefore, often received several cross-match fees from the same unit of blood. The pathologists who ordered supplies of blood from the Red Cross and allocated them among patients had little incentive to avoid outdating since the Red Cross charged a fee only for units transfused.

The cost of outdating was borne entirely by the nonprofit Red Cross, while much of the control over outdating resided with proprietary hospital labs. As I was concluding my study, the Red Cross changed its policy, shifting a large portion of outdating costs over to the hospitals. When part of the outdating cost was shifted to the hospitals, as far as I was aware the hospitals did not in turn shift part of that cost to pathologists through renegotiation of contracts.

The proposition that the assignment of hepatitis liability to nonprofit hospitals and blood banks would lead to an optimal transfer of risk to attending physicians through a bargaining process seems to be open to question. Low transaction costs may not be a sufficient condition where some of the parties are nonprofit and others proprietary. In any case, to the extent that full liability succeeds in reducing hepatitis, it loses its effectiveness as an economizing incentive; that is, where part of the risk is borne by the attending physicians, the greater the reduction of hepatitis resulting from the liability placed on blood banks and hospitals, the smaller the increase in the physician's incentive to economize on blood transfusions.

The evidence presented in the testimony of Dr. Okuno to which Professor Havighurst referred is somewhat puzzling. This evidence was given to support the impact of the *Cunningham* decision. This decision held an Illinois hospital strictly liable in a case of post-transfusion hepatitis. Dr. Okuno, in his letter, presents evidence that doctors practicing in a nearby hospital subsequently became significantly more efficient in allocating blood to patients. However, there is nothing in his letter that explains how part of the hospital's risk was shifted to the physicians. In evaluating this evidence, it is important to determine how the physician's incentives, as distinct from the hospital's, were affected by the *Cunningham* decision.

AUDIENCE PARTICIPATION
AND DISCUSSION

PROFESSOR GORDON TULLOCK: This question is essentially for Professor Havighurst. You referred only to civil law, but why not also to criminal law? Clearly, a person who says he has not had hepatitis in order to get a $50 fee for donating blood has committed fraud in a perfectly traditional way, and it seems possible that he is guilty of murder if somebody dies as a result.

It might well be that prosecuting attorneys could deal with this problem, particularly since the man who has had hepatitis does not know whether it was B or not and hence does not know whether it will turn up in the tests immediately. At least at the beginning, a fraudulent donor would have an even chance of going to jail, and there might be a sharp reduction in hepatitis.

PROFESSOR HAVIGHURST: I have never heard of a case of that kind, but the theory is as you stated it. If the form filled out by the donor indicated that criminal liability for homicide could attach to an untruthful statement concerning the donor's experience with hepatitis, one might find a dramatic change in the behavior of paid donors.

PROFESSOR DONALD MARTIN: I have two remarks, one for Professor Havighurst, the other for Mr. Hurst.

First, it appears that there is some misleading analysis here—misleading in the following sense. We see different statistics coming from the United States and from England. From the United States, we see a high incidence of serum hepatitis compared with that in Great Britain. Professor Havighurst says we must examine strict liability as a means of imposing costs on those who would supply blood. I am not in disagreement with that particular remedy. However, one must also ask what is the liability rule in England. Are we really saying that we can explain this differential between the United States and England—a differential that is, at least implicitly, a challenge to our system—by differences in liability rules? Are there differences in the liability rules of the United States and England?

PROFESSOR HAVIGHURST: My understanding is that there is no rule of strict liability in England and that the frequency of suits of this kind in England is considerably lower than it is here, so whatever incentive effect such suits might have would be minimal in England.

PROFESSOR MARTIN: My second remark is to Mr. Hurst. You mentioned that when you, as an outsider, look at the data you find that more people are standing up to give blood every day. There are donors out there, altruistic or otherwise, who want to give blood. Is it not the case that there is in some sense a chronic shortage of blood? And by shortage I mean that the amount demanded is greater than the amount supplied at the current price for blood. Are you not faced with a chronic shortage of blood?

MR. HURST: No, we are not faced with a chronic shortage. By virtue of the fact that we are dealing with an item of limited shelf life, with occasional wide fluctuations in demand and with some demand for extremely rare blood, even a prudently run blood program may experience temporary shortages. Viewing the blood situation of this country in total, such shortages are infrequent and certainly not chronic.

PROFESSOR MARTIN: Okay, there are no great blood drives, for example, urging people to donate. Do most people volunteer simply by walking into blood donor centers?

MR. HURST: Oh, no. I am not suggesting that in any way. There is a highly motivated group of people working in the nonprofit blood sector who are constantly encouraging people to donate.

I am aware that blood has been imported into the country, but we can find isolated cases to prove any point that we try to make. I reiterate that in this country there are no chronic shortages, and that, on balance, there is an adequate supply of blood to meet legitimate medical needs.

PROFESSOR MARTIN: So there is an effective zero price for blood except for the commercial market. Let us suppose that the market is in two sectors, the nonprofit market, which relies on zero-price donors, and the paid market. Can we say that in the nonprofit market, the amount we want is there at any moment we want it?

MR. HURST: I think you are trying to bait me. Obviously, there is no magic to making donors appear—it takes hard work and lots of it. There are substantial numbers of trained professionals in donor development communicating the need for blood and stimulating the public to donate. This is not without cost to society. The difference is that the donor receives no direct remuneration.

TED MILLER: I would like to raise three points. The first concerns Dr. Okuno's letter. It appears that the period in which he said his major changes occurred was the period in which the popular press, particularly in the Chicago area, was publicizing the problems of hepatitis. He may have confused the power of the press with the power of the law in his analysis.

My second point concerns strict liability. From the viewpoint of economic equity, liability makes sense. Certainly, by permitting physicians in the hospitals to insure themselves and to pass the cost of insurance on to the end recipients, the cost of hepatitis will be spread more equally across all people who receive blood. But, conversely, because of the additional cost of legal action, the average cost of blood will be increased. Currently, when we do have a liability suit at all, it is against the doctor or the hospital.

Somebody could conceivably sue the doctor, the hospital, the blood center, the company that supplied the blood center with its blood packs, the company that supplied the blood center with its labels, and some other people in the middle. Now, many of those people might not actually be liable, but it is a very common practice, especially in auto liability, to sue a whole chain of people. Defense against that becomes very expensive.

My third point concerns the questions of cost and economic efficiency. There is a question whether the volunteer or the commercial system is more efficient and cost-effective. It must be remembered that long before there was a question of hepatitis, long before there was any onus on commercial blood from the viewpoint of safety, approximately 80 to 85 percent of the blood collected came from volunteers. There is a lesson to be learned there.

A more important issue for the economists is that, at least here in the United States, we have two basically different philosophies of what a volunteer donor is: one philosophy accepts individual responsibility, and the other accepts community responsibility. In the case of individual responsibility, a replacement fee is frequently imposed, creating a completely different supply curve and demand curve in that there are two prices for the blood from a blood center. The question of whether the individual or community concept of a volunteer is more efficient may be a more important economic question than the question of commercial versus volunteer.

DR. JAMES CRISPIN: I would like to ask Mr. Hurst if one of his negative comments about commercialism is not a positive one. He cited the lack of scientific advancement and research among commercial blood banks. I am the medical director for a profit-oriented, commercial plasmapheresis center and, in collaboration with ethical pharmaceutical houses, I have written extensively in this area. In fact, every major practical scientific breakthrough in the field of blood banking in the past ten years, in my opinion, has been a result of commercialism. One example is the advent and the use of RH-immune globulin, which is produced in our commercial plasmapheresis establishments and is fractionated by ethical pharmaceutical houses. The hepatitis test itself and the first 300 liters of anti-hepatitis antisera used in this first-generation test were produced at my own center by plasmapheresing positive donors. And so it goes, right on down the line. The fact that we have large quantities of livephiliser factor 8 to treat hemophiliacs in this country is a result of commercialism. In fact, England is now importing this factor because its volunteer system has failed to keep up with the need in Britain. Other examples are gamma globulin and fibrinogen, as well as the plastic bags with separate compartments that are in virtually universal use today, which are all the result of our commercial blood system in this country. And even the typing serus; we hyperimmunize people to produce anti-A, anti-B, and anti-D, and so forth. Without the commercial sector, blood banking would be in the dark ages. If we had depended upon the research and development of the volunteer system, through the Red Cross, for example, would we have any of these things? I seriously doubt it.

MR. HURST: I would like to make one point, and that is that I had hoped in the introduction to my remarks to indicate that I was making a broad generalization based on personal opinion and observation. Very obviously, there are exceptions to that, and certainly the remarks that you make show a glowing example of a great contribution coming from the commercial sector. I was generalizing, and my apologies to you, again, if I overlooked any of your contributions.

PROFESSOR TULLOCK: One of your generalizations was to dispute my point that good intentions are not enough, and it appears we have heard a refutation of your generalization. If you would like to withdraw it—

MR. HURST: Good point. In view of the evidence that was presented, I certainly would qualify it.

ARTHUR CARROLL: I would like to ask Professor Havighurst if he would respond to the suggestion that donors be prosecuted for fraud and that people then be given the option of deciding whether they wanted the blood.

PROFESSOR HAVIGHURST: I am always sympathetic to the line of argument which says that consumers ought to be given a choice as to what to take and what not to take and how to spend their money. But there are times when the process gets so detailed that consumers are unable to make very effective choices, and this is such a case.

It is unrealistic to expect the patient to be given a clear choice and to exercise it sensibly. One might impose a rule of strict liability and then allow the patient to elect a different regime. This is very roughly the Epstein thesis, which I find interesting, though with the reservation that it is easy for the medical profession to overreach patients in this way. For example, if the medical society should develop and make available a standard form whereby patients waive their right to recover and if nearly every doctor in town used that form to change the rule of law, I would have objections. On the other hand, I do not object if one patient and one doctor discuss the matter at some length and agree that they will operate under a different legal regime. I guess the rule of strict liability is where we should start.

PROFESSOR ROTTENBERG: I am not convinced that the contractarian solution is the right one either, and I remain open to argument. Perhaps Mr. Havighurst will explain what is so different about blood? Consumers do not know very much about elevators either. And, indeed, if elevators are of low quality, there is damage to the public health. Consumers do not have much knowledge of the physical properties and capacities of plumbing systems, and if they do not work that adversely affects the public health. There are numerous products that adversely affect the public health, but we permit consumers to buy them.

PROFESSOR HAVIGHURST: The rule of strict liability or something close to it applies to many of those products now. The important point is that the caveat emptor notion is widely regarded as antediluvian where dangerous products are involved, yet it applies to blood, which is one of the most dangerous products around. I find that peculiar. Now, while caveat emptor is a doctrine that is dying, it will never die completely, because there are many things on which the courts would rule that consumers assume risks and can be presumed to do so knowingly. We would agree that the courts ought to attempt to draw that line, however difficult the task.

My general view of the entire problem of malpractice might shed some light on the discussion and some of the comments. Previous speakers, particularly Professor Reddin, have referred to me as if I were a spokesman for the American Trial Lawyers' Association, but I certainly am not. (The ATLA represents the plaintiff lawyers of America.) Both Mr. Reddin and Mr. Levine appear to identify me as a spokesman for the legal profession and as an advocate of more jobs for lawyers, and a number of people have referred to the high costs of the tort litigation system, which I apparently am thought to advocate.

Actually my preference is implementation of an insurance system with the objective of strict liability based on a no-fault principle. This system would not require the filing of lawsuits but would provide compensation automatically. I have written about the malpractice problem and have largely rejected the fault system as it now exists. I have proposed instead switching to no-fault insurance, using experience rating to keep providers conscious of the costs that fall to their patients.

The matter is complex. My articles are cited in the footnotes to my paper. I also made reference at several points in the paper to my preference for a no-fault insurance system and to Professor Franklin's proposals for an insurance system. Since insurance normally reduces the lawyer's role, my critics mistakenly assert that I think lawyers have a great contribution to make. I am, however, proposing that law, statutory law if necessary, can make a contribution in defining responsibilities, but I need not defend that proposition at great length.

There are costs involved in shifting losses even through an insurance system, and we have to be certain that the costs of shifting losses are justified by the benefits derived. For many losses of the kinds that we encounter in the area of medical malpractice—post-transfusion hepatitis being one of them—I am satisfied that shifting the loss to the providers, that is the blood banks and hospitals, in some way would be highly beneficial.

Regarding Mr. Wargon's question of who ought to bear the costs, my thought is that the kinds of bargaining that I would like to see occurring between doctors and hospitals is indeed difficult to bring about. Mr. Wargon apparently has evidence that such bargaining seldom occurs, but in the no-fault scheme that I propose for malpractice the assignment of risks to one party or the other—the doctor or the hospital—would generate bargaining. Each party would have something to give that the other wants. For example, the surgeons would ask the hospital to change its behavior by hiring nurses who can count well so that they will not leave sponges in incisions after surgery. The hospital might agree to hire better sponge counters if the surgeons would be more circumspect in the use of blood and not use it simply to restore color to a patient's cheeks after surgery. The bargaining that would be generated would be precisely what we have always wanted the medical system to undertake—namely, better interaction between doctors and hospitals looking toward improving the quality of health care.

DAVID ENNIS: Let me respond to Professor Rottenberg's question about the difference of blood. But first, a suggestion for Mr. Levine and the Food and Drug Administration. I suggest that FDA require a label for all speakers on blood bank solutions warranting that they have been fully responsible for procuring blood for a blood center over a period of six months and, second, that they have given blood within the last twelve months. I view the noncritical, self-satisfying, cosmetic decision to buy a car with a roll bar as substantially different from the life-and-death decision by a physician that a blood transfusion is required. The timeliness of the transfusion and the availability of the product (if you will excuse the term) complicate the decision beyond the simple acquisition of a material thing.

PROFESSOR ROTTENBERG: The point is interesting, but I think it is wrong. I said blood is not different from many other products, and I meant that it is not different in one respect—that is, there are many products that cause adverse side effects with some positive probability. Indeed, products appear in a kind of an array. The probabilities of adverse side effects are high for some models of that product and low for other models. This is also true with respect to occupational tasks. One is more likely to encounter black lung disease among workers in an underground coal mine than in an open pit mine. We permit people to make choices in the selection of occupational tasks and in the purchase of products when, in fact, they may choose high-probability adverse-side-effect products or adverse-side-effect models of both occupations and products.

My question with respect to blood was, If you permit individuals to make decisions about these products and occupations, why not permit them to make decisions about the quality of blood they purchase? In that sense, I do not see anything special about blood. One could design a social policy that sets some bottom limit to the risk the consumer is permitted to purchase; for example, one could prohibit people from buying anything or engaging in any occupational task if the probability of an adverse side effect of some magnitude is higher than 4 percent. If you choose, as a matter of social policy, to do that kind of thing with respect to blood, then you ought to choose it with respect to all other products.

By the way, the roll bar in automobiles is not cosmetic. It is intended to prevent the top of the car from crushing if the car rolls over. It is a safety feature. I still do not see what is different about blood.

MR. REDDIN: Briefly, I am not sure if anything has happened to the distribution of income in the United States since I was last here, but one of the implications of what Professor Rottenberg suggests (making varying qualities of blood available at varying prices) would rather imply that the poor, as usual, will get the rotten stuff. Has the distribution of income so changed in this society that people can make real choices about the quality of the blood they receive rather than having it determined by how many dollars they have in their pocket?

MR. CULYER: I would like to discuss briefly what Mr. Rottenberg said. In an area where so many people are so sure about everything, it is ironic to pick on Rottenberg, who is a good skeptic, but he is skeptical with regard to some things that surprise me.

Reuben Kessel's evidence was—if I recall it correctly—that the opportunity cost avoided in terms of treating hepatitis cases amounted to something like $156 per unit of blood. That is, on the average, high-quality blood saved $156 of hepatitis-related costs. Now, that suggests that high costs of collection, if they must be incurred to ensure safer blood, may be—in some social cost-benefit sense—worth incurring. Pursuit of high-quality blood may not be forcing "society" to pay a higher price for blood than "society" wishes.

The other issue he raised was the question of the proper attitude to risk. It would be extremely presumptuous for us to assert that absolute risk aversion is the policy that ought to be adopted, but individuals do appear to be, in fact, extremely risk averse in this particular area. Hence, a public policy couched in terms of minimizing the risk of hepatitis is probably as near to the social optimum as one could get. It does not follow, however, that strict liability is the only way of doing this. In the United Kingdom we do not have this system, and we do not have a commercial system.

Although there is some evidence of periodic shortages and postponed operations, in Britain we have fewer shortages and lower incidences of hepatitis and we probably have lower waste rates (whatever that might mean) than you have in the United States. So, clearly, strict liability is not the only way, but, given the general nature of the U.S. market, it may be more appropriate than the United Kingdom's administrative solution.

PROFESSOR HAVIGHURST: I would like some clarification of Mr. Levine's original statement. He cited Titmuss for the proposition that we should seek the lowest technically possible risk of hepatitis. Then he seemed to imply that the Food and Drug Administration had adopted this as its policy, meaning that it is willing to impose costs of $156 per unit, or thereabouts, on blood suppliers. How certain is the FDA that its regulations do, in fact, improve the quality of blood? Is that settled, or do these requirements simply sound good on paper? Have they been validated by comparing costs and benefits?

My concern, as I said in my paper, is that a market system based on roughly correct incentives and without a centralized system to decide who will do what and how often is perhaps more reliable because it allows people to adapt to circumstances. In particular, they can omit doing things that do not pay.

MR. LEVINE: The justification for various regulations is objectively verifiable. For example, the Food and Drug Administration has recently required hepatitis testing at the third-generation level of sensitivity. Unquestionably, the required RIA testing will screen out more potentially dangerous units of blood with the B service antigen than the previous second-level test. Other regulatory requirements are established as a result of rule-making procedures based upon published proposals, which provide for public comment, always very extensive, before the promulgation of a final order. I have yet to see a final order that is promulgated as it was originally proposed. The system is designed to elicit all available data for consideration in the decision-making process. In any particular case, whether or not the government judged wisely between divergent data will always be subject to debate.

PROFESSOR TULLOCK: Titmuss said and Mr. Reddin repeated that the existence of a commercial blood market prevents people from making gifts. I have never been able to understand that. Suppose I buy a pint of blood from Mr. Martin, here. I fail to see how that act prevents anybody else from giving a pint of blood. I have heard this charge repeatedly, but I have never heard an explanation of it. Could you elaborate on this point?

MR. REDDIN: I have not asserted it so bluntly today, but I have argued that, when the two sectors exist side by side, they will interact. That relationship can work in several ways. For instance, individuals in a city with two blood agencies, one a giving one, one a selling one, might interrelate. I can envisage that these sectors might survive separately, unrelated, not influencing one another, if the city were neatly segregated socially—in other words, if the sellers lived in the inner city and the charity givers were out in the suburbs. Neither would use the other as a reference group.

But, if the donors and the sellers do refer to one another the situation changes. The fact that I can go to one place and get twenty dollars for my blood and go to another and get "nothing" for it might well affect my decision about where to go. But most important, it might discourage me from giving altogether if I thought that someone—an intermediary—was making a profit from my gift.

My concern with the existence of the commercial market is not just its impact as a competing purchaser, but also its role as intermediary or handler of blood products. The presumption that someone will make a profit out of my gift would certainly discourage me from giving. If I possessed a highly superior moral sense and still felt strongly about the need to give my blood, then perhaps I would not mind if a profit-making intermediary were ripping somebody off for handling the stuff.

PROFESSOR TULLOCK: Suppose that I was a bad businessman and regularly losing money on my commercial blood bank, so there was no profit. Would you object to giving to my bank? (By the way, nearly half of all business firms in this country are in this situation.)

MR. REDDIN: That is possible. I am making these assertions not as fact but rather as my own responses and those of other donors. In Detroit a few years ago, some donors told me that they gave to one agency rather than another because of the efficiency and cost characteristics of those agencies. Many of them said they had chosen the Red Cross because they thought it was efficient and had lower costs than commercial blood banks. They saw that what they gave would be passed on to the recipient as a gift. That is small-scale, unsystematic evidence from a single area. But I certainly do not see this as such an unreasonable thesis; it is entirely possible that donors look for some efficiency in the intermediary handling of their gift.

MR. CULYER: The trouble with that view is that to somebody with sufficient imagination anything is conceivable. The interesting question is, What actually happens?

DAVID EISENMAN: For ten years I tried to get some student involvement in blood banking in Champaign-Urbana, Illinois. We finally got the local blood bank to agree to accept pints which would be assigned to specific patients without charge to the patient. It must be stressed that these donations are not insurance

85

for the donor's family. They are donated on behalf of someone who has already received blood, for forgiveness of the replacement requirement or the responsibility fee. We signed up a number of students, who were typed and then put on a waiting list. Three years after these students were typed, the student who had led the effort was asked to give a pint. He went to the hospital, gave his pint, and then was offered twenty-five dollars. He told them he was a volunteer donor and was giving blood on behalf of some needy person who had received a transfusion. He was told, however, that the hospital had no mechanism for that, and that if he gave up the twenty-five dollars, the hospital would simply keep it. There was no way it could transfer a credit to an unspecified person.

Today in Illinois there are blood banks that operate on a replacement fee or a contractual arrangement of the kind Mike Reddin has described. If someone has given a pint to cover his family and offers a second pint to someone in the hospital who has received more than five pints and is having a hard time replacing them, he will be told that his donation can be credited to any family he names, but there is no mechanism for transferring that pint to an unspecified individual. What is a donor to do when he faces that kind of situation?

PROFESSOR TULLOCK: I find it strange that the people in Illinois cannot figure out that giving the twenty-five dollar fee to a needy sick person is the equivalent of giving him a pint of blood.

MR. EISENMAN: How can it go to a specific person?

PROFESSOR TULLOCK: By asking the hospital to put that twenty-five dollars toward someone's bill.

DR. CRISPIN: Mr. Reddin said something that, once again, I am unable to pass up. He characterized volunteers as being in the carriage trade and commercial donors as being from a lower socioeconomic class. This raises a question for Mr. Levine of the FDA with regard to mislabeling. As we know, many college students donate blood for money. The Red Cross has also, within the past few months at least, drawn blood from donors in prisons. Prison donors have a much higher incidence of hepatitis than college students. Nevertheless, the Red Cross would have to label blood drawn from prisoners "volunteer blood" while the commercial blood obtained by paying college students would have to be labeled "paid donor—high risk." Would this constitute false and misleading labeling on the part of the Food and Drug Administration?

MR. REDDIN: Yes, it would. I have not drawn the distinction between a paid and a volunteer donor in that way. I recognize the distinction as a function, if you like, of socioeconomic status coupled with the risk factors identified by Dr. Gocke this morning. The fact that there are middle-class student blood sellers

86

does not negate my argument at all (although it may tell us something about students). The commercial donor population is *typically* characterized by the inclusion of high-risk donors of low socioeconomic status—I did not deny that there were a few transient exceptions to that generality. I simply focused on the contrast between the downtown unemployed male and the suburban housewife in order to make the point.

But my conclusion runs counter to the general tenor of the participants' comments so far. If we want as many as possible to give, then the blood-collecting agencies should not immediately dash out to the suburbs and leave the downtown donor to sell his plasma or rot. We should not reject and isolate the poor from giving in their society. We should pursue a policy of enabling them to participate.

Necessarily, this policy choice must be made first, and research objectives will flow from it. I want to be able to cope with and incorporate the high-risk donor. We should identify the high-risk donor not to screen him out, but rather to do something for him, to keep him in. This is why, to my mind, research in "blood-washing" techniques is such a critical area—it enables us to use the product of the disease-carrying donor (as, of course, we do already in the preparation of antigens, and so on). With this overriding policy objective, to include rather than exclude, we do not pursue a flight to safe suburbs and safe donors— we use agencies that go to the prisons as well as to the churches, to skid row as well as to the executive suite. Since both the United States and Britain have excluded the poor from so many options, let us not cut them out of this one as well.

DAVID WILLETT: I address my question to Professor Havighurst. I understand your suggestion that strict liability is intended to ensure better quality care rather than to compensate the patient; presumably the cost to the patient of the injuries sustained is already being met through his own disability or hospital insurance. Previously, this kind of liability was the subject of insurance. Therefore, the liability damages were not borne by any person or entity who could obtain insurance against civil liability. But we are faced with a situation now where liability is limited to fault or negligence and general liability insurance is becoming practically unavailable. Do you really believe that insurance is going to be available to blood banks, or are you suggesting that this liability not be insured but be borne by the blood blank or the hospital? Is that a tolerable situation?

PROFESSOR HAVIGHURST: It would improve insurability if liability were limited in some way. It is a debatable point in itself, however, whether or not any pain and suffering damages, for example, would be payable. Liability could be determined on a formula basis so as not to involve a jury. The liability likely to be found in a particular case would be defined. If the hospital or blood bank were required to provide first-party insurance to the recipient of the blood that they supply, there would be a relatively predictable risk, and insurers would be able to write a policy that would cover it. The problem of predicting future claims and awards, which has threatened to destroy the availability of malpractice insurance, would not be great.

MR. WILLETT: At least are you suggesting that, under the present rules of allowing unlimited recovery, we could not afford this strict liability that you propose?

PROFESSOR HAVIGHURST: Professor Franklin, who has written about this issue at considerable length, appears to prefer the Cunningham approach and use of the tort system. He suggests the insurance system as an alternative to be considered. The insurance system would be preferable, but it is not essential. Once the legal rule was clear, cases would be routinely settled. Insurance availability for this event would be no problem.

PROFESSOR WARGON: I have a question for Professor Havighurst concerning insurance. How would the insurance be designed so that the hospitals, blood banks, and physicians would still have some incentive? That is, how would some part of the loss still fall on them as a result of hepatitis?

PROFESSOR HAVIGHURST: Premiums would be set in accordance with the hospital's experience over time. The policy might also be designed with a deductible or some kind of copayment requirement so that the hospital would, indeed, recognize a cost to itself from every case of hepatitis that occurred among its patients.

It would be important, of course, that Blue Cross or Medicare not pick up the premiums actually paid as a reimbursable cost. There is a risk, of course, that the government and Blue Cross would not recognize the desirability of leaving that incentive feature intact.

It is also important to recognize that we do not have a closed system. The way we sell medical services, with insurance paying most of the costs of medical care, makes patients able, even though they might not be willing, to pay very high prices for slightly improved care or reduced risks. There is, therefore, a risk that introducing incentives would induce excessive spending on safer blood beyond the optimal point where marginal benefits and costs were in balance. Consequently, it would be unnecessary to impose the full costs of any hepatitis case on the hospital. As long as the hospital recognized some significant cost to itself, there would probably be enough incentive to determine ways in which it would lower hepatitis incidence.

PART TWO

DOES GOVERNMENT REGULATION WORK?

DOES GOVERNMENT REGULATION WORK?

Harry M. Meyer, Jr.

The Regulatory Mechanism and the Swine Flu Virus

It might surprise outsiders to know that at the Food and Drug Administration we occasionally ask ourselves: is what we are doing worthwhile and does regulation work? It might not occur to you that some of us do worry about those things. We may not do much about them, but we think about them. In this context, I thought it might be useful to take an offbeat approach to the regulation of blood by the Bureau of Biologics, namely, to examine it from the perspective of the bureau's very recent activities pertaining to the swine flu virus. If I were a swine flu virus, what would I think of this ponderous government apparatus? Is it really cost-effective in denying me my proper place in the lungs of people? Since all of you have developed very definite opinions about the myriad government regulations in general and those affecting blood services in particular, I thought it might be refreshing to examine the government versus swine flu as a test case through which we can perceive the usefulness of regulation. I do promise, however, that I will take off my gloves and swing directly at a few blood issues as well.

One can think of a flu virus as a ball covered with surface antigens, but the frustrating thing about flu viruses is that they are always mutating and changing those surface antigens. Whenever that surface changes, it is a new surface to us, and, if we are not immune to the new antigens, numerous bad things may happen. Frequently, they do.

If one goes back to 1918, 500,000 deaths in the United States and 20 million around the world were caused by the swine flu. The Asian flu epidemic of 1957 was caused by the same virus with a totally new surface. That epidemic swept the country killing nearly 70,000 Americans; it depends upon which statistician's figures one accepts as to how many people actually died. This past spring, we had a visitation from a very slightly different flu virus called Victoria. As a consequence we had a little bit of flu that killed 20,000 Americans. This was what is called a medium-grade flu epidemic, which is nothing special unless one happens to be one of the 20,000.

What does the government do in these cases? Well, the first factor concerning us is the detection of new viruses. The U.S. Public Health Service and the World Health Organization conduct detection systems: they swab throats, check diseases, and try to detect new flu viruses as rapidly as they occur in the population. As they detect such viruses and discover how different they are from familiar types, how widely they are occurring, and what the pattern seems to be, an attempt is made to define the risk to the population from that particular virus and to determine the appropriate precautions. Does one launch a massive vaccine program? Or, at the opposite extreme, does one ignore the virus? These decisions must be made by the government.

Then we come to the question of economy. Economists frequently think that the private sector should have a free say in doing things, and I am a good private-sector man myself, particularly when I pay my taxes. But government is necessary for flu-vaccine programs. In 1957, when a new virus with new characteristics popped up in Hong Kong and posed a real threat to this country, our detection system worked well, and we decided vaccination was necessary. At that stage, what happens? We inform the manufacturers, who examine the facts and wonder whether people will buy vaccine. The drug manufacturers must decide on the amount of money to gamble on the vaccine and the speed with which they should move. They do move, but they are gambling. If a manufacturer places $10 million or $20 million into vaccine production and nobody buys the vaccine, what is to be done with it? Should it be poured down the drain? There is a real risk factor here.

In the fall of 1957 manufacturers produced about 50 million doses of vaccine. Then the public, in its infinite wisdom, began being vaccinated on the recommendations of the government, the doctors, and other medical authorities. About half of the vaccine produced—25 million doses—were actually innoculated in people. Shortly thereafter, however, the Asian flu appeared to be easing a little, and the public not to stick its arms out. Consequently, approximately 25 million doses of vaccine ended up on the manufacturers' shelves and were never used for innoculations. Unfortunately, however, the flu kept occurring. We had a big flu epidemic after Christmas, and 30,000 people died. I think we can agree that this was not an effective program. I cite it to show the limitations of an untouched market system in which there are no guarantees: no guarantee that what is produced will be purchased and no guarantee on attempts to deliver vaccine to the population.

Now I would like to turn to other aspects of the government's role in working with industry to produce a vaccine. After the Public Health Service and scientists have detected a new virus and have tried to define the risk it implies, the government provides the manufacturers with seed viruses. The government provides many "candidates"—strains from here and strains from there—in the hope that one or two of them will prove to be the ideal candidates from which to produce a vaccine. Subsequently, the manufacturers become heavily involved. They must adapt the virus to the growth of eggs. They must obtain, in the case of the swine flu program, which attempted to make vaccine available to everybody, perhaps 100 to 200 million eggs. They must gear their production systems to work seven days a week and overtime in order to deliver enough vaccine with a minimum of errors. The government tried to insure that the swine flu vaccine would be produced at the maximum rate of speed by making a contract, with money furnished by Congress. The contract guarantees the purchase of massive doses of the vaccine and thus nearly eliminates the financial risk of the manufacturers.

Another element that the government becomes involved with is clinical trials. A new vaccine cannot suddenly be given to 200 million Americans. Clinical studies must be carefully designed, with many variations and doses, to insure that the vaccine will safely produce a protective antibody response in the various population groups receiving it, including infants, pregnant women, and the very old. For the swine flu program, these clinical trials involved the Public Health Service, the federal government, and some 6,000 men, women, children, and old people who were innoculated. On the basis of the trial results the government is able to advise industry of the precise dosage and recommend how each group should be innoculated.

Even then, government's role is not over. The regulatory organizations and pertinent government agencies must coordinate and control the quality of the vaccine, just as they control blood banking. Government is involved in testing, along with the manufacturers, and in releasing individual lots of vaccine as they become available to be certain that their quality is evenly maintained. The government is also involved in evaluating what happens to people who receive the vaccine. What reactions will occur and, if the flu does occur, how much protection will be provided by the vaccine? All these activities require government interaction with the private sector.

The *New Yorker* of May 31, 1976, carried an article entitled "Swine Flu over the Cuckoo's Nest" which began:

> History was made last week at the Annual Academy Awards night, when, for the first time, a single disease captured virtually every major prize given by the prestigious American Academy of Medicine. The Swine Flu Virus, a relatively unknown pathogen, whose last starring role was in 1918, carried off coveted Jonases for best disease, best symptoms, best virus, best potential epidemic and four other categories.

One of those "other categories," I feel sure, must have been the best case for government intervention. Without massive federal involvement at many stages, the private sector simply could not wage a war against swine flu.

The History of Blood-Market Regulation

I hope I have convinced you that regulation does work to some extent, at least with viruses. Let us turn our thoughts now to the regulation of blood services.

The federal regulation of blood and plasma began in the 1940s when it was appended to the existing biologics regulatory apparatus of the National Institutes of Health. The mission of NIH is research, and the orientation of biologics regulation, in the many years when it was controlled by NIH, reflected this view. Referring to the then infant national blood program, the director of NIH wrote in 1968: "The direct responsibility of the NIH in this program ends with the development of technology and a demonstration of its application to existing problems in the blood field."

In July 1972, the biologics regulatory component of NIH was transferred to the Food and Drug Administration, Bureau of Biologics. The creation of the Bureau of Biologics was more than a simple change in the organizational chart and title. The most important change may have been the conveyance of the regulatory mission from a primarily research-oriented organization, NIH, to the FDA, which was historically concerned with the compliance aspects of regulation.

Because biologics and drugs were for the first time brought within the jurisdiction of a single agency, the provisions of the Food, Drug and Cosmetic Act and the Public Health Service acts that, prior to that time, had been used for biologics were now administered by a single group without jurisdictional confusion. The effects of the transfer were quickly realized both inside and outside the bureau. At least four primary actions have been taken in these past several years that give an overview of the interaction of regulation.

First was the development of regulations. Any compliance program is dependent upon three elements: (1) the basic legislation outlining the area of regulatory control and the limits of the regulating agency's authority, (2) court decisions interpreting both legislation and regulations, and (3) the promulgation of regulations in the *Federal Register*. The regulations serve to define the standards for preparing the products, and their publication provides a legally sanctioned method for eliciting input from industry and from many parts of society.

Only six products were regulated and codified by the Bureau of Biologics at that particular time. There were three blood-bank products, whole blood, red cells, and cryo-precipitated antihemophilic factors; two derivatives, immune serum globulin and measles immune globulin; and one diagnostic product, the antibody associated with hepatitis. Other products, such as donor plasma and normal serum albumin, were subject to so-called minimum requirements that had not been published in the *Federal Register*. These requirements were similar to guidelines. Many of them had not been revised or changed since 1949.

To remedy this deficiency, the Bureau of Biologics initiated a concentrated effort to update and revise the minimum requirements in the Code of Federal Regulations and to solicit comments from the public sector to be considered in developing more formal standards. A second area that received attention was the regulation of intrastate blood banks. Blood banks that ship blood for interstate sale had been licensed for a number of years under the Public Health Safety Act, but intrastate blood banks had not been regulated. The regulation of intrastate blood banks comes firmly under the jurisdiction of the FDA via the Food, Drug and Cosmetic Act because blood is a drug as defined in the act. Therefore, all establishments engaged in the preparation of blood, blood components, or blood derivatives were potentially subject to the Kefauver-Harris Amendment of 1962 and to the requirement that drug establishments register with the FDA. This is the basic authority, then, for FDA's regulation of intrastate blood banks. All registered intrastate establishments are subject to at least biannual inspection, and the far-reaching implications of the drug statutes apply to all blood banks except those that serve solely the blood repositories. As a result of this successful move to bring the intrastate banks under the general umbrella of the FDA, the bureau's oversight powers, which had previously affected 126 licensed establishments, were extended to affect over 7,000 facilities dealing with blood products.

Because neither act authorizes the delegation of inspectional obligations to nongovernmental bodies and because few of the state health departments had blood-bank inspection programs, the responsibility for carrying out inspections of intrastate blood banks has been assigned thus far to the FDA field investigators. Full implementation of that broad new inspectional program, however, had to await two other developments. One was the publication of additional standards for some of the regulated products, the other the publication of the so-called Good Manufacturing Practices (GMPs). With the publication of these GMPs on November 18, 1975, and their implementation a month later, formal intrastate blood-bank regulation began.

A third major area of FDA blood regulatory activity pertains to source plasma. Largely as a result of market and technical factors, the plasmapheresis industry rapidly evolved as a separate force within the biologics area, but it was not placed under regulation by the federal government prior to 1972. In order to ensure uniform standards of operation and adequate protection for donors, the Bureau of Biologics undertook an ambitious and rather aggressive program to regulate the plasmapheresis industry in 1973.

Standards were published dealing with source plasma as a definable product, with plasma collecting and processing, and with the manufacturing of other injectable products. All manufacturers of source plasma were notified that their products would be subject to license effective January 1, 1975. During 1974, the bureau reviewed and conducted prelicensing inspections of 250 applicants and suspended operations in about 80 establishments that were in violation during that early period. Since January 1975, four plasma establishment licenses have actually been revoked, in contrast to the revocation of only a single blood-bank license during the past thirty years. This suggests that it was more difficult to raise standards by regulation in the plasma industry than in the blood-banking industry. In May 1976, source plasma regulations were amended to include all source plasma that would be used for any purpose, not only that used for fractionation.

Hepatitis is the last of what I consider the four separate definable areas in which we have been involved. The Bureau of Biologics has been said to be preoccupied with hepatitis. The most notable expression of the Bureau of Biologics' preoccupation with hepatitis was the requirement that all blood and plasma collected for transfusion or for further manufacture be tested serologically for the presence of the hepatitis B surface antigen. Since December 1975, all such testing must be done by the third-generation method, which is the most sensitive of the available methods. Results from a number of sources have convinced me that there has been a considerable reduction in post-transfusion viral hepatitis due to hepatitis B that is in good part related to the advent of sensitive hepatitis testing.

The bureau's concern has, however, been manifested in a number of ways besides hepatitis testing. With the Good Manufacturing Practices, we have insisted on uniform standards. This creates a climate in which all personnel become acutely aware of the various snares in their craft and the problems these can cause. While the GMPs and hepatitis testing will not in themselves eliminate hepatitis, their use has certainly reduced it. The first four years since the creation of the Bureau of Biologics have seen the establishment of the regulatory ground rules by which the blood community is operating. In general, their effects have been beneficial.

The Future of Blood-Market Regulation

What is the next four-year plan? (I do not say five-year plan, because I know some people feel that would identify me for what I really am.) Turning to the future, I think I can identify a few highlights that are of particular interest.

Plasmapheresis is not dead. It is like a snake. You keep stamping on it, but it keeps coming back. Plasmapheresis and plasma supply and demand and related matters continue to generate international as well as national debate. Prior to our regulatory offensive, there was—and this may not be widely known—a drain of plasma from developing countries into the United States to supplement our domestic supply. The economists in the audience would call this a negative trade balance. With the rather strict regulation that has taken place in the last two to three years, we have virtually stopped importing plasma. Today nearly all the plasma in this country comes from plasmapheresis establishments located in the United States. Indeed, after fractionation much U.S. plasma supplies the European market. This fact, which is beyond regulatory jurisdiction, has been a subject for considerable public comment.

Now we have a positive trade balance, and some say that we are bleeding American donors dry in the process. Others, with a keen interest in, for example, the cost of hemophilia treatment, say that the exportation of plasma is maintaining a higher than necessary price for antihemophilic products in the United States. This issue ties in with the question of social versus individual responsibility for, say, hemophilia carriers. Some states have legislated in this area. The question of paid versus voluntary plasmapheresis, too, remains. I am not proposing that we should adopt an all-voluntary plasmapheresis plan, but again I note that this is an issue that is being discussed.

Some time in the future Congress may take a stand on one or more of these plasma-related issues. Which course it will adopt remains to be seen. Predicting the behavior of Congress is not much safer than predicting flu virus mutation.

We are examining the problems of overlapping jurisdictions among our regulations affecting blood banks. In order to retain some measure of local control and yet respect the intent of the various laws, the bureau has carried on a dialogue with the blood community in the past year with the thought of developing an experimental program designed to license not only individual blood establishments but entire regional systems. Under the regional licensure concept, a core collecting facility and its hospitals would be granted a single umbrella license. This plan could be implemented without additional legislation, but we believe it needs further discussion before it is implemented. As most participants in this conference know, the Bureau of Biologics is also working with groups in the American Blood Commission who are investigating regional concepts in their search for progressive ways of dealing with regulatory issues.

The bureau has an interest in blood data collection. We, like most people, are convinced that an evaluation of the performance of the blood-service complex has to rest on the evolution of a detailed, realistic, and quantitative data-collection system and set of performance criteria. Most are aware that we have finally, with a lot of consultation over the last year or two, started a system called Blood Inspection Establishment Registration System (BIERS), which is now beginning to collect data. I hope that within the next year or two we, working with those in the blood community and in the American Blood Commission who are interested in data collection, will be able to determine the feasibility of this system.

I have left blood labeling to last. The Illinois Blood Labeling Act was passed in August 1972—about the same time we joined the Food and Drug Administration—and shortly thereafter, we asked the general counsel of FDA whether we could develop labeling rules under our existing statutory authority. A number of other developments were also occurring at that time. We had just introduced mandatory hepatitis testing in blood banks, the radioimmunoassay test was just coming forward for licensure, and the concept of non-A, non-B hepatitis was being discussed. That was the period when we were all looking and thinking and, even though we got legal approval for labeling from our general counsel, we elected to wait. We thought it would be reasonable to wait while Illinois was developing experience with its labeling law. Specifically, we wanted to determine the effects on the blood supply of the Illinois labeling act. At the same time, we contracted with the New Jersey State Department of Health to work with us in collecting hard information about the nature and significance of many risk factors connected with post-transfusion hepatitis and to determine which of these factors might be subject to manipulation.

The results of the studies were summarized in the *Federal Register*.[1] In this proposal we stated that there was a fairly clear relationship between hepatitis incidence, the prevalence of hepatitis antigen, and blood collected from paid donors. The reduction of hepatitis in the state of New Jersey was fairly substantial when there was a reduction in commercial blood from 36 percent of the total supply in 1969 to about 9 percent in 1973. By September 1975, it was pretty clear that in Illinois labeling had produced, so far as we could see, no major supply problems. A similar California law was soon to become effective, and many other state legislatures were discussing labeling laws.

As we summed up the three-year results that we were accumulating, it seemed that hepatitis B antigen testing had been fairly effective in reducing the incidence of post-transfusion hepatitis due to hepatitis B but not at all effective for A. In fact, by that time we knew that hepatitis A was not particularly important as a cause of post-transfusion hepatitis. But we also knew that there was a non-A, non-B hepatitis, which was an important health hazard. It, too, occurred more frequently after the use of commercial blood than after the use of volunteer blood.

By this time, every major nonprofit blood-banking organization, including the ABC, was on record as favoring an all-volunteer blood system. In retrospect, I think some would probably conclude that the bureau was, if anything, rather sluggish in drafting a proposal for blood labeling. From the discussion prompted by the original proposal published in the *Federal Register* we learned that some of those not-for-profit blood banks were probably not as keen on an all-voluntary blood system as their public statements indicated. Some of the government's economists may also have learned that the public's perception of barter and trade in human tissues departs slightly from economic theory.

We all recognize that labeling will not totally solve the post-transfusion hepatitis problem. It will not come close to totally solving the problem. But labeling, in our best judgment, would help inform the physician and the public of the hepatitis risk and lead to changes in blood procurement and use that would substantially reduce the occurrence of transfusion-associated hepatitis.

Where does the blood-labeling proposal stand now? Following the evaluation of the many comments received from the blood-banking community and a review of the transcript of the open meeting that was held at NIH on March 18, 1975, we are digesting the views and information we have and licking our wounds. The bureau will publish a reproposal defining the terms "paid" and "voluntary" donor some time this year. Comments on the definitions in the reproposal will then be invited from the public.

---

[1] *Federal Register*, vol. 40, no. 221 (November 14, 1975), p. 53040.

Summary

After my comments today you may still ask if I believe that the regulatory process works. Each of us has an independent streak in his nature; we all react somewhat negatively when someone intrudes upon what we are doing. When the Government Accounting Office looks over my shoulder, I become restless. Even those who are the most doctrinaire in this regard, however, generally recognize that drugs, like death and taxes, unavoidably require some regulation.

Churchill's often quoted remark about democracy—that it is "the worst possible system except for all those other systems that have been tried from time to time"—sums up, in a sense, some of my thoughts on regulation. As a man on the inside of the skunk works, I regard the FDA with considerable misgivings, more than you might suspect. However, I do not see any solid alternatives to FDA regulation, or at least any alternatives that offer any greater promise. Nevertheless, those of us who are on the inside of regulatory organizations should try to remain attentive to the public and to the suggestions of professional and public groups. We do try our best to listen, because it is extremely important to be prepared to change any time somebody can make a persuasive argument for a different case.

Allow me in summary to say that we regulators are frequently shot at and we are frequently hit. Anything we do or anything we do not do makes somebody mad. Being an engineer at heart, I like to remember one comment that John Kennedy made, when he said that his experience in government was that when things are noncontroversial and beautifully coordinated, there is not much going on. In the blood field there must be an awful lot going on right now.

PART THREE

CURRENT PRACTICES
AND SUGGESTED REFORMS

CHAIRMAN'S COMMENTS

John J. Corson

The prominence of blood in the array of services provided by the nation's health-care delivery system has become increasingly evident. This prominence is due to advances made in blood-banking techniques, surgical procedures, and the therapeutic application of blood. It derives, in addition, from the fact that blood transfusion is the most highly developed form of human tissue transplantation. I might add that a third reason for the singular attention being given to blood is that, in many respects, the policy and organizational modality represented by the American Blood Commission—the implementing of public policy through means devised by the private sector—indicates that deficiencies in at least one part of the health-service system can be alleviated through the collaboration of consumers and health-care providers, without government regulation.

It is proof of the importance of the issues related to blood that individuals representing a wide range of professional and consumer interests gathered to discuss them under the auspices of the American Enterprise Institute. The issues surrounding the collection, processing, distribution, and use of blood are sufficiently complex and novel to generate considerable interest and controversy. As a result, studies of the attitudes, decision processes, and behavior of blood donors, as well as discussions of sociological principles, economic models, the locus of legal liability, and the systematization of performance measures are brought to our attention.

One of the more intriguing aspects of blood services is indicated by this level of interest and controversy. If regional interaction among blood-service facilities becomes a guiding framework for the coordination of services, I believe we will witness a more optimal use of technical resources and a more efficient and appropriate distribution and utilization of the supply of blood. As the discussions and audience participation at this conference revealed, there is far from a consensus as to how blood should be collected and distributed, how the expenses of blood services should be met, what kind of service units should be involved, whether proprietary organizations seeking profits should be permitted to participate, how much concentration of control and participation should be allowed or encouraged,

103

and so forth. In such a setting, the constructive interaction of economists, legal experts, social scientists, and medical scientists and practitioners is a welcome and necessary ingredient in the resolution of problems. Through such measured and deliberate consideration we can receive guidance for the future development and improvement of the performance of the nation's blood-service community.

GETTING PEOPLE TO GIVE BLOOD: SOME IDEOLOGIES, PRACTICES, AND ISSUES

Alvin W. Drake

In this presentation I shall consider some of the issues associated with whole-blood collection in the United States. Much of what I have to say is opinion and interpretation. This is not a presentation of research results.

My comments deal only with the *supply* side of the blood service complex. Following a few introductory remarks I wish to discuss six topics: (1) one way to characterize blood-collection ideologies, (2) some phenomena that tend to make the practices of blood-collection systems more nearly alike than their ideologies, (3) several elementary considerations that pertain to the comparison of blood-collection systems, (4) my research and its objectives, (5) a personal interpretation of the "blood-supply problem," and (6) the sets of blood-collection issues that I believe to be of primary importance.

The blood supply in this country is composed of two major sectors. The sector most visible to the general public consists primarily of the collection of whole blood intended for transfusion and for transfusion components. The dominant collectors of this part of the supply are hospitals, community blood banks, and the Red Cross. This supply will amount to something in the order of 12 million units this year, drawn from a total of about 8 million donors. Accurate figures are difficult to obtain. The rate of growth of this supply is often estimated to be in the vicinity of 10 percent per year.

The second part of our national blood supply is thought to be larger in volume and much of it is drawn by plasmapheresis from what is believed to be a much smaller set of donors. These collections are made primarily by large pharmaceutical companies or their agents and are used in large part for plasma and for products derived from blood. Most of my presentation is not concerned with this sector.

It is obvious that the total blood supply constitutes an important aspect of the health-care system. However, we have astonishingly little data of the type that might allow us to estimate the degree to which medical practice is constrained by blood supply. Concerns with hepatitis transmission, the availability of blood, and several other developments have directed considerable attention to blood during the 1970s. Some of these developments are not necessarily the result of shortcomings in the blood supply. A few of the developments are merely anecdotal, and some, of course, arise from organizational differences among the large collectors.

Several of the developments which helped bring the blood supply into the limelight are:

(1) The Titmuss book, *The Gift Relationship*, arguing that the blood supply in the United Kingdom, by virtue of its all-volunteer nature, achieves levels of purity and availability far better that those achieved in the United States. Some arguments of social policy and their implications were very clear to Professor Titmuss. With the important exception of hepatitis rates, he found little reason to obtain any significant data on the strengths and weaknesses of the blood supply in the United Kingdom.

(2) Several television documentaries, one of which included an unforgettable scene of outdated blood being poured down one of the least attractive sinks in the state of California. (This is comparable to revealing that firemen are often sitting around fire stations rather than fighting fires, though it would probably occur to many people that firemen should be available when homes and businesses do, in their unpredictable ways, catch fire.)

(3) A growing interest in the reform of the blood-supply system in Congress and in the Department of Health, Education, and Welfare. It is this interest, along with the interest of senior professionals in the field of blood banking, that resulted in the creation of the American Blood Commission. Some people may consider the interaction of the government with the blood-supply industry a test of a particular mode of government intervention in the health-care field. (This mode, I would say, consists of lots of attention, some—probably little—self-improvement prompted by the threat of legislative action, occasional harassment, and limited dollar investment.)

(4) Robert and Suzanne Massie's book, *Journey* (New York: Knopf, 1975), relating the experiences of a family determined to compromise as little as possible of the lifestyle and opportunities of a son who has hemophilia. The book includes some comparisons of the blood services the family encountered in this country and in France. Although the book received much attention, I think the press generally overlooked what I consider to be the authors' primary message, namely, that the problems they describe are endemic to the way health care is delivered to patients with chronic needs in this country, whether or not those needs center on blood and blood products.

(5) A proliferation of articles in the popular press, often of a sensational nature, providing the general public with reasons to be terrified about the quality of the blood supply. Typically, such articles described an experience with the drawing

facility of a commercial firm and implied, at least by omission, that this is the source of the blood one would be likely to receive in a local hospital.

(6) Increasingly strong documentation showing that blood purchased from donors, coupled with inadequate control of the paid-donor population, can provide a very high rate of hepatitis transmission. (The best laboratory tests are believed to be able to detect the disease in only about half the units of blood that carry it. The major collectors of whole blood have made large reductions in the amount of blood purchased from donors during the last few years.)

This list could be much longer. A large number of bills pertaining to the blood supply have been proposed in the Congress. My intention has been only to note some of the relevant developments. These developments focus attention on the blood supply, but in themselves they generally do not provide useful assessments of actual problems nor do they help us gain perspective on the relative importance of different problems.

After this general and oversimplified introduction, I would like to attempt to sort out some of the ideological issues associated with blood collection.

Characterization of Blood-Collection Ideologies

Blood collection involves a number of practices and notions, such as assurance, credits, insurance, nonreplacement fees, coverage, predeposit, and individual and community responsibility. It may be helpful to use a simple framework to characterize blood-collection *ideologies* and to separate them from particular practices. Thus, in this section we shall be concerned only with ideologies. Theory and practice are very different, so do not be surprised if you have difficulty relating your own donation experiences to the issues we are about to discuss.

For most purposes, we need only the answers to two simple questions to specify the underlying ideology of any blood program. Although finer distinctions among ideologies are possible, they seem to me to be of considerably less importance than these.

Question 1: Community or Individual Responsibility? There are several ways to state the first of our two questions. A common, but not adequately specific, form of this question is: Is it the responsibility of individuals or of the larger society to ensure that blood will be available when individuals need it? We use the following nomenclature for the two possible answers to this question:

Community responsibility (CR). After blood is collected, it is distributed for use as common property of the entire community. With regard to their own blood needs, donors receive no considerations of any kind different from those provided to nondonors.

107

Individual responsibility (IR). It is the responsibility of individuals to make some arrangement to provide for their own potential or actual blood needs.

The two answers differ sharply with regard to the connection between a person's participation in the provision of the blood supply and the situation the person encounters as a patient. CR requires identical considerations, in every way, for patients who have and for patients who have not given blood. IR allows (and CR does not allow) a coupling between a person's contribution to the blood supply and some aspects of the situation that arises when the person needs blood. An IR blood program might include arrangements such as (1) requests for the predeposit of blood before admission to a hospital for elective surgery, (2) blood-credit systems of various types, (3) recruitment of the family and associates of the patient for blood replacement, (4) the utilization of recruitment messages indicating that donors and their associates will be subject to certain advantages in time of need, and (5) the assessment of charges ("nonreplacement fees") to patients who have no provision for replacing (with blood or blood credits) the blood they have used.

There are several ways that advocates of the two ideologies argue their beliefs. CR advocates may think it essential that conditions be identical in every way for all people at the time they require something as unique and precious as blood. Advocates of IR may think it improper not to offer at least some limited blood-related advantage to people who make provision for the contribution of something as unique and precious as blood.

Question 2: May There Be Exchange between Blood and Money? My second question for the specification of the ideology of a blood-collection program requires less explanation: May there be an exchange between blood and money at any point in the blood-supply system? Although the meaning of the question is obvious, it is difficult to differentiate sharply between the two possible answers. We use the following nomenclature for the answers:

Special gift (SG). Blood is a special gift which may never be bought or sold. It should never be exchanged for money or for anything that can be converted into money. Donors should never be given money for their blood and patients should never pay money for blood itself.

Market commodity (MC). Blood may be bought and sold. The market price reflecting the value of blood may be recognized in monetary as well as in other terms.

Although it will not matter for our discussion, I should admit that I know of no entirely satisfactory way to define "anything that can be converted into money." (Personally, I would label SG a system in which employers allow employees to donate blood during working hours. The point can be argued either way.)

An MC system might purchase blood from donors, have a nonreplacement fee, or have blood-credit programs in which the premiums may be paid in money as well as in blood. An SG ideology would not permit any of these practices.

If it seemed useful, we might make a further distinction between the two points at which blood and money could be exchanged in an MC system. Although I believe this distinction matters primarily because of its practical rather than ideological consequences, some people might argue that paying donors is ideologically different from charging people for blood they cannot replace.

The two questions presented in this section, with only two possible answers allowed for each question, provide us with enough of a framework to discuss ideologies and their relationships to actual practices in a relatively explicit manner. First, in order to become more familiar with the notions discussed here, let us look at one example of each of the four resulting fundamental ideologies: CR-MC, CR-SG, IR-MC, and IR-SG.

Examples of the Four Fundamental Ideologies. Under some system ideologies, such as IR-MC, one could design a wide variety of blood programs. Even in an (unusual) case where all blood-collection practices are entirely consistent with a system's ideology, many choices remain in the selection of the particular arrangements under which a blood program is to carry out its operations.

This section will present one example for each of the four ideologies that result from our classification scheme. Many alternative examples could be provided. For these examples, I shall not provide all of the more obvious assumptions for each case.

Example of a CR-MC system. Consider a nation which purchases its entire blood supply from citizens who choose to sell their blood. Let this be a nation that provides blood free to all patients under a system of socialized medicine. The ideology of this system is designated CR because all aspects of the treatment afforded donors and nondonors with regard to their own blood needs are identical. The MC part of the ideology follows from the fact that there is an interchange between blood and money, which happens, in this case, to relate to the purchase of blood from donors. If some of the blood supply were given freely and only a part of it were purchased but other conditions remained as stated above, the system in this example would still be designated as having a CR-MC ideology.

Example of a CR-SG system. Consider a state in which only volunteer blood is collected from donors and in which no benefits are assigned to the donors. Thus, this is a state with no credit systems and no nonreplacement fees in which patients and their associates are subject only to the recruitment efforts directed at all members of the general public. Again, the ideology is CR because no aspect of a patient's situation relates to whether or not the patient has contributed in some way to the blood supply. The SG designation indicates that there is no interchange of blood and money in this system.

Example of an IR-MC system. Consider a region in which the blood supply is provided by "donor clubs," groups which pay a collective premium in blood donations to cover the potential blood needs of club members and their families. Nonmembers who require blood are asked to arrange to replace the blood, and, if they cannot do this, they are charged a nonreplacement fee for each unit of blood used. This example has an IR ideology because, when patients need blood, the situation is different for members and nonmembers of the donor clubs. The MC characterization of the system's ideology accounts for the fact that, in some circumstances, a patient may be required to pay for blood.

Example of an IR-SG system. Consider a region, such as the one above, where blood is raised by donor clubs to provide for the blood needs of members. Assume that nonmembers with blood needs are asked to make efforts to pre-deposit or replace blood, but the alternative of paying a fee instead of providing blood (or blood credits) does not exist. Nonmember patients are subject to recruitment requests that are not made to donor-club members when they need blood. Because it does not present identical conditions to all patients at the time they need blood, the system is IR. It is SG because it does not allow for any interchange of blood and money.

These hypothetical systems illustrate four "pure" ideologies that can be defined through the answers to both of our questions. There are a few additional comments I would like to make to conclude this section.

There are problems with defining the jurisdiction of blood systems. These jurisdictions may be geographical regions or sets of people, and it is easy to think of situations in which a person might be subject to several systems or caught between them. A little more will be said about this problem later. I would also make the point that, when one considers the blood-collection systems in other countries, one discovers no consistent match between a nation's political ideology and its blood-collection ideology. A list of the blood-collection ideologies of other countries often surprises its readers. It appears that blood supplies of excellent quality and economic efficiency may be possible under each of the four ideologies we have defined.

Practices Are More Similar than Ideologies. Essentially every blood program has a stated ideology. This ideology is most visible at the highest administrative levels. It is a simple matter to match the stated ideology of any particular blood program to one of our four "pure" ideologies. I call these ideologies "pure" because many considerations intervene between theory and practice in a blood program. This section considers some of the phenomena that make the practices of different blood programs more similar than their ideologies.

Especially from the point of view of a patient who uses blood, several concerns do depend on the ideology of the local blood program. Such potential concerns include costs and replacement pressure. I suspect that there are a considerable number of blood programs, however, in which the general public, the donors, and sometimes even the patients would have difficulty in describing either the ideology or the practices of their local blood programs.

Let me list five of the factors that tend to homogenize blood-system practices, whatever the underlying ideology may be.

(1) In all but the most unusual circumstances, the *availability* of blood for a patient with immediate needs is unrelated to the patient's blood coverage and financial situation. In the United States, this is true under all ideologies. (There may be important exceptions, however, for some people with chronic needs.)

(2) In a system with a CR-SG ideology, it often happens that the people with front-line recruiting responsibility deliver recruiting messages with IR implications, hinting that some aspect of the situation when one needs blood is better for those who have given than for those who have not. Furthermore, CR-SG systems may attempt to "personalize" their operations by taking steps such as asking donors "in whose name" they would like to make their donations, even though a CR-SG system may do nothing whatever with the information after it has been obtained.

(3) Whether they are developed by IR or CR blood collectors, all the mass media blood messages I have seen deliver similar information to the public. These communications tell the public something about the need for blood and about where to donate. Although some may exist, I have never seen any mass media announcements that present IR argument for donation. By implication, the announcements present CR reasons for donation.

(4) IR groups usually generate a blood supply for a community considerably larger than the membership whose supply is assured by the group. In systems where there is no nonreplacement fee and nonmember patients are exposed to little or no replacement pressure, we have a program which is essentially CR-SG but which recruits donors under an IR-SG banner.

(5) Some hospital employees and physicians, aware as they are of the value of blood and the dangers of not having it, may feel compelled to approach patients and their visitors about the importance of replenishing the blood supply. This is one more possible source of IR practices in CR systems.

We have noted some of the forces that make blood-program practices more similar than one might expect from the program ideologies. In CR systems, some front-line activities may take on an IR flavor. A donor moving from a region with

111

an IR system to a place with such a CR system would be unlikely to detect the difference. In any case, it is probably easier for an IR system than a CR one to keep its practices consistent with its ideology.

Some Considerations for the Comparison of Blood-Collection Systems

Discussions of blood policy eventually lead to the evaluation of alternative blood-collection systems. We require bases for the comparison of blood-collection ideologies and of the practical consequences of implementing these ideologies. I am certainly not in a position to suggest a framework that allows such comparisons to be made in a convincing and meaningful manner. I do wish to comment on some elementary considerations that apply to such comparisons, however, and to warn against oversimplified comparisons.

Bases for the comparison and evaluation of blood systems seem to group themselves into three somewhat overlapping areas—economic, medical, and ideological. Most people would agree that the medical bases are the most important. These three areas are discussed here in order of increasing difficulty.

Because of the multiple products, services, and potential clients associated with a single unit of blood, the economic analysis requires sophisticated accounting and remains subject to several interpretations. Even when the economic analyses are performed by professionals with adequate resources and backgrounds, open questions remain (for example, are we concerned with the cost of a unit of blood to the patient who receives it, to the patient who may receive it, to the collector, or to the entire society?). From my own limited knowledge, I see no reason why any one of the four ideologies should perform with greater economic efficiency than the others.

If there are reasons why a particular ideology might be preferred on economic grounds, the reasons would arise from practical aspects of its implementation rather than as direct consequences of the ideologies themselves. As has been observed many times, for example, it does not necessarily follow that volunteer blood is acquired at a lower cost than purchased blood, nor does it follow that the presence of a nonreplacement fee necessarily contributes to the economic efficiency of a blood-collection system.

The medical bases for comparison have several aspects. Two of the major concerns are the quantity and medical quality of the blood supply achieved by various blood-collection systems. Again, these measures are likely to relate more to the details of actual practices than to the ideologies themselves. Other medical issues are concerned with the relative merits of the ways that different blood-collection systems distribute donors among the population. It is possible that, when implemented, some ideologies produce systems that tap a small core of donors frequently, while others draw blood less frequently from a larger set of donors. One might argue that the former arrangement imposes a slightly higher risk on its donors and a higher degree of quality control on the resulting blood supply. The latter arrangement, relying upon less frequent drawing from a larger population, seems to provide a more promising base for the future expansion of the blood supply. These issues become important, for example, if there is truth in the conjecture that CR systems tend to obtain fewer, but more frequent, donors than is the case for IR systems.

An additional medical issue for the comparison of blood-collection systems is the forming of judgments on the medical desirability of large central collection programs and facilities to support higher technologies of blood therapy. This concern seems less relevant than others to our present discussion.

Finally, the ideological (or "moral") bases for the comparison of blood-collection systems are the most difficult to discuss. It is at least possible that a large collection of people could agree on suitable economic and medical measures of system performance. A person's selection of the most important ideological issues (and related topics, such as "measures of fairness") will be much more dependent on the person's background and responsibilities. The emergency physician, the recruiter, particular members of the general public, the patient, and the sociologist may choose to emphasize very different aspects of blood-system ideology. I shall merely sample the breadth of the total set of moral concerns we may expect to find.

An emergency physician may emphasize the need to use all reasonable approaches to see that blood needs are met. The physician's primary concern may be the availability of blood when and where it is needed; he may be far less concerned with either the ideology or the practical details of generating the blood supply. The sociologist, more or less at the other end of the scale, is likely to be concerned with what, in his view, blood-banking practices say about the nature of a society. The emergency physician may see sociological theory as somewhat remote. The sociologist has no patients who require a transfusion of a rare type of blood around three o'clock in the morning.

Ideologies with regard to blood donation also vary, of course, among members of the general public. Just as there are people who believe it is ideologically wrong to give a donor anything or any advantage in return for a blood donation, there are people who believe it is ideologically wrong *not* to extend some special consideration in return for a person's willingness to give blood. (My own work indicates that most people, including donors, have had little reason to think about this issue. What people say is strongly influenced by whatever they are told by their local blood-collection system.)

As one last example of the variety of views to be considered in attempting to evaluate blood programs in ideological terms, consider the situation of a clinic which purchases a very high-quality blood supply from a small donor pool and does so without creating problems for other health-care facilities. Perhaps the purchase arrangement is believed to be the most reliable and effective way for the clinic to obtain type-specific fresh blood precisely when it is desired. Staff members may argue that any changes in their blood-collection policy that are likely to lower the quality of their blood supply are obviously immoral, no matter what the ideology behind the changes.

It is clear that large ideological differences exist and will continue to exist, even among professionals who are highly informed about blood banking and entirely committed to the quality of the blood supply. It seems unlikely that the underlying issues are subject to complete resolution by any scientific or analytic process, even if we had reliable measurements of the various systems' performance.

When, for example, the emergency physician and the sociologist disagree, assuming that both of them are reasonably well informed, it seems foolish to think of the issue in terms of who is right. Rather, I see their conflict as defining the need for some type of social decision process such that most parties may accept the decision process itself as a fair one and are likely to be able to live with its results. The question who is to decide for whom may not be omitted from any list of ideological considerations.

In concluding this section, let me note several points with regard to the ideological considerations that enter into a comparison of blood-collection systems:

(1) It is easy to make forceful, oversimplified comparisons. This is done all the time and often serves only to further polarize the major collectors.

(2) Although many individuals have strong preferences one way or the other, it can be argued that both CR and IR are deeply rooted in the "American way of life," both within and beyond our health-care system.

(3) The most critical measures of blood-collection-system performance, such as the redistribution of risk, health, and costs, may depend far more on the details of actual system practices than on system ideologies. Even if it were the case that practices were entirely consistent with a system's stated ideology, we see no compelling reasons why one particular ideology should outperform all others.

(4) In any useful discussion about blood policy, it is important that people appreciate the variety of ideological viewpoints held by other people.

My Research Work

Supported by a grant from the National Center for Health Services Research, I have been trying to learn about public attitudes and decision processes with regard to blood donation. I am also interested in the training, working environments, incentives, and modes of operation of people who have professional responsibilities for donor motivation, recruitment, and retention. In large part, it is the experience I have had with this project that gives me the courage (or the nerve) to attempt the general interpretation of the state of the blood supply that I will now present.

Although it is unbearably slow and often a clerical nightmare, my fundamental source of information has had to be survey research. The sets of respondents with whom I and my students have worked include:

(1) samples of "frequent donors" in four metropolitan areas,

(2) samples of "apparent ex-donors" in the same four areas,

(3) samples of delegates to the Central Labor Bodies in four cities,

(4) samples of the general public in three cities,

(5) sets of high school students at about the time that many of them encounter their first convenient opportunity to give blood, and

(6) a few working units in large companies. (By studying this group we can compare donor and nondonor perceptions in a situation where the availability of blood-donation opportunities is about the same for all participants.)

The survey work is designed to help us develop models of how, in the course of their lives, people form their attitudes and make their decisions with regard to blood donation. We are interested in issues such as people's perceptions of various collection agencies, attitudes toward blood policy, knowledge about blood and perceptions of the need for blood, and the particular circumstances in which people become donors and ex-donors. A primary concern is the need to understand the attitudes, knowledge, and decision processes of the large part of the eligible population that has never given blood.

Pretesting our survey instruments, identifying the types of information with the greatest potential value, and making the organizational arrangements to allow some of the survey work to be performed have taken a long time.

I believe that this project is the first effort of its kind to be performed in a consistent manner in a variety of different blood-collection environments. Our studies with controlled samples of the general public in three metropolitan areas, along with similar studies of captive audiences in a few large insurance companies, allow consistent comparisons between donors and nondonors.

The field work for this project was completed in June 1976. A great deal of the analysis remains to be done. An overview of the work is to be presented at the AABB annual meeting in the fall of 1977.

The remainder of this section presents examples of a few of the things we are learning. This is clearly an informal and very incomplete overview. All of the results indicated below are approximate. All are subject to important qualifications which relate to the samples used, the response rates achieved, and, of course, to the incomplete state of the analysis.

Studies of Frequent Donors and Former Donors. In cooperation with centralized blood-collection programs in four metropolitan areas, we have been working with "frequent" and "former" donors. Frequent donors are people who, by the standards of their local blood programs, have been making donations relatively frequently. For the purposes of this research, a former donor is any person whose most recent donation was made twenty-four to forty months prior to the survey. There are, of course, considerable difficulties in identifying and contacting people who appear to have stopped donating.

Contrary to the folk wisdom of the blood-banking field, ineligibility and bad donation experiences can account for no more than about 25 percent of the former donors among our respondents. Our survey instrument sought assessments of the most recent donation experience and its effect on the respondent's willingness to donate again. We also inquired about changes in health and attitude since the most recent donation. The only item that provides a significant separation between the former donors and the frequent donors is the respondent's perception of a regular solicitation and a reasonably convenient donation opportunity. The former donors and the frequent donors do not differ significantly in terms of their estimates of the need for blood or their attitudes with respect to blood policy.

Three of our survey locations are primarily IR-MC and one is CR-SG. It was interesting to find that the former donors at all four locations are similar in almost all regards, including demographics and donation histories. Former donors, as well as frequent donors, have a very favorable view of the collection agencies to which they made their most recent donation and of the treatment they received at that time.

Comparisons between the frequent donors at the three IR sites and the frequent donors at the one CR site are unreliable. We do not know whether some of the differences we have identified relate to blood-program ideology, to the operational practices of our one CR system, or to other factors. The relatively frequent donors in these IR systems donated considerably less often than the relatively frequent donors in the CR system. (If we assume the per capita blood collections are about the same at all locations, this may suggest that the IR systems achieve a broader donor base.)

As might be expected, although it is not at all indicated in the existing literature, donors in the two types of systems express reasons for donation and sentiments about blood policy that very much reflect what the donors have been told by their collection agencies. For example, frequent donors in the CR programs believe that assurance and insurance plans would not help them in their personal efforts to recruit new donors. Frequent donors in the IR systems believe that assurance and insurance programs provide a vital incentive in trying to recruit new donors. Blood-collection agencies almost surely play the leading role in determining people's attitudes about blood donation and blood policy.

Incidentally, I was surprised to learn that most frequent donors believed that they have never been asked to recruit new donors. This was true at each of the four locations.

Studies of the General Public. Our survey work with the general public has been conducted in three metropolitan areas—Hartford, Houston, and New York. As a rough estimate, it appears that about 40 percent of the people presently in the age bracket for blood donation in these three metropolitan areas, taken as a whole, have given blood at least once. About 25 percent of the people in this age bracket believe they are ineligible at the present time.

Among people who have never given blood but believe they are now eligible to donate, we consistently find little evidence of a particularly strong reluctance to donate blood. Given the obvious limitations of methods that ask about attitudes rather than observing behavior, this issue is pursued in several ways. People are asked to indicate, in their own words, their best understanding of how it is that they never happened to make a blood donation; they are asked to assess the importance of reasons why some people do not give blood; they are asked about the likelihood that they would give blood under particular sets of circumstances, and so on.

Of our respondents who believe they are eligible now but who have never given blood, only about 15 percent agree with the statement, "I have made a relatively firm decision *not* to be a blood donor." About 5 percent of these people responded that they are not sure whether they agree or disagree; the remaining 80 percent disagree with the statement.

These and many similar results suggest that the majority of eligible non-donors have never been pressed very hard to think through their attitudes and behavior with regard to blood donation. In my view, it has not yet become necessary to press these people very hard or to confront them with realistic donation opportunities because, in most places at most times, their blood is not yet needed to achieve an adequate supply.

Finally, we do not find important differences between donors and nondonors in many areas where we might expect such differences to occur. By and large, for example, donors and nondonors do not differ much in their perceptions of the general need for blood, in their estimates of the chance that a typical person or hospital patient will need blood, or in their attitudes with regard to blood policy, such as how they feel about cash payment for blood. In some cases where differences are found, the differences may reflect natural differences between the two classes of respondents (donors and nondonors).

A Personal Interpretation of the "Blood Supply Problem"

All discussions of blood policy make a large number of implicit assumptions about the present state of the blood supply. At this conference, some of us may state views of the situation more explicitly than the data really justify to allow the comparison of assumptions and to encourage further discussion. Although my own research does substantiate some of what I am about to say, it would not be correct to assume that I have (or that anybody has) a solid basis for views on all of the following matters. Nevertheless, the discussion is significant. One's views on blood policy are likely to depend a great deal on how one assesses the present blood supply in the United States.

With such provisos, I suggest the following interpretation of the present state of the blood supply:

(1) In most of the country, at almost all times, the blood supply performs at a remarkably high level. The blood-services complex provides a level of service so high that a great many physicians and surgeons pay little more attention to the blood supply than to the water supply.

(2) The blood collectors are among the few organizations that appear to believe, in several ways, that they and the blood supply are well served by being slandered in public. Very few programs go out of their way to make the public aware of the quality of their blood services and of the adequacy of the supply they provide. Many collectors believe that public response is best when the public believes more blood is badly needed to reinforce an apparently marginal supply.

(3) The primary constraint on the total level of blood collections is the actual level of medical need in the area served. Collectors appreciate the need to maintain a responsible level of collections and, although they could often do so, they do not overcollect.

(4) The second major constraint on the total level of blood collections is associated with the resources and organizational skills of the collectors. In areas with several major hospitals, coherent community blood programs appear to be vital for the achievement of adequate and effective blood collections. Community-wide programs can approach large employers and groups, as can public education programs, much more successfully than programs sponsored by individual hospitals.

(5) At least at the present level of collections, we cannot find signs of a major reluctance on the part of the American public to give blood. (This may change as demand grows in the future and might change if we were to increase voluntary collections to try to meet plasma needs.) The reason "so few people give blood" at the present time is that the donors now active are the number required to provide an adequate blood supply. In starker terms, I would argue that the primary reason more people do not give blood is that the whole-blood collection system does not need their blood at the present time. If we had had a 20 percent increase in the number of donors last year, giving at about the existing average donation rate (about 1.5 donations per donor per year), all parties con-

cerned would have been embarrassed by the resulting outdating figures. Similarly, I believe that there are large untapped populations of potential donors in essentially all communities. In part, these populations have not been reached yet because their blood is not really needed yet.

(6) There certainly are problems in ensuring a balanced and timely, predictable supply throughout the year. This does not require *more* donors as much as it requires more resources and management skills for the collectors. The working habits of most collectors contribute to our seasonal shortages at least as much as do the working and donation habits of the American public.

(7) At the present level of the need for whole blood, there are no clear indications that blood-collection ideology relates directly to the adequacy of the resulting supply. Committed professionals (and I have yet to meet a recruiter who describes his work as "just another job") working under any ideology or blend of ideologies, with adequate organizational resources, appear to meet needs well. Ideologies may affect donor profiles (slightly) and the distribution of donors in the general public, but they need not affect either the quantity of blood collected or the cost and difficulty of collecting it. There are innumerable trade-offs among the practical consequences of ideologies (replacement provides a very personal approach but it may not produce frequent donors, CR may tend to produce a small core of very active donors, IR may attract the widest donor base and elicit administrative services from donor clubs, and so on), but it is not at all clear that there is a need for the selection of a common blood-collection ideology on a national scale.

(8) There is great danger in describing the blood-supply system as a unified one with similar and severe problems throughout the country. There may be a few critical geographical areas in which major organizational changes are required to develop an adequate blood supply. This situation does not, in itself, justify major intervention in large areas where, by whatever means, an excellent level of blood service is already provided.

(9) None of the above comments should be taken to imply that all is fine with the blood supply. Patients, especially those with chronic needs, may be subject in some places to conditions the American public would not knowingly accept. It is important to realize both that this problem is not unique to the blood services and that, as the system is now constituted, many of the problems of people with chronic needs relate to products that are not always provided solely by the blood banks or hospitals.

These are my personal conjectures on the present state of the blood supply. By making our assumptions explicit, we have a better chance of understanding each other's position and of directing our attention to the most important issues.

Some Present and Future Issues. To further encourage discussion, I would like to identify five primary sets of important issues on the supply side of the blood-services complex. In their approximate order of importance, beginning with items of highest priority, are the following sets of key issues:

(1) *Assessment of the supply.* For all the awful things said about the blood supply, often by its own professionals, we have only incidental evidence (with the possible exception of hepatitis rates) on whether the blood supply significantly limits the delivery of medical care. Such information can come neither from outdated figures nor from a few lurid stories. It must come from the professional users of the supply (the physicians) with the assistance of blood-banking officials. A national assessment would probably indicate that (1) the whole-blood collection and distribution system itself is generally far better than the utilization of blood and (2) overall supply problems exist only in a limited set of geographical locations. Such locations may merit the most attention, especially in the formulation and professionalization of responsible central collection agencies.

The main part of my proposed assessment would be an attempt to determine the degree to which the present blood supply affects the selection and timing of medical procedures. The primary information source would be the physicians who select and perform the procedures.

(2) *Chronic needs and larger gifts.* A very important set of issues deals with the plasma supply, services to people with chronic needs, and the development of workable procedures to encourage an appropriate level of larger gifts, such as those we ask of the plasmapheresis donor. The underlying policy issues, including the allocation of scarce resources to chronic users and the interplay between public and commercial collectors, seem so difficult that we tend to bury this topic. As blood technology improves in the future, this set of issues will grow larger and more central.

(3) *The degree and style of government interaction with the blood services.* As much as possible, the motivations of federal actions should be stated, the evidence on which the actions are based should be stated, and the actions should be consistent with the stated motivations. A dedicated official in a first-rate blood program might continually sense very generalized attacks on the blood-service community, some of them unbalanced enough to be based less on documented shortcomings than on ideology. Although intervention based on both may be warranted, it should be frankly identified for what it is. We want the best blood services that can be provided. But it may not be productive to "require" levels of performance in blood services that may be an order of magnitude above our most ambitious hopes for many equally important and far less-developed aspects of the health-care system. Beyond a certain point, it may not be reasonable to ask the blood-supply system alone to attempt to resolve incredibly difficult issues

of policy and redistribution, both of which are currently in much worse shape in most other parts of the health-care system.

(4) The integrity of blood-collection messages. Some time in the future, it may become important to consider the integrity of some of the blood-collection recruiting messages delivered to the American public. If this does not receive adequate attention soon, I believe the issue might eventually lead to a crisis with regard to public confidence in the blood collectors. Perhaps in the name of the "greater good," blood is often collected under premises that are marginal and possibly false.

All blood-collection systems must affect the transfer of blood from healthy people to people with blood needs. This message is rarely conveyed to the public, although the newer blood technologies are likely to make it even more important in the future. More and more donations will be required to supply the needs of people who cannot provide blood. Recruiting messages are usually put in other terms. And rarely is the public told it has an excellent blood supply or asked to maintain it. Because of the types of recruiting messages that often do appear, serious problems could arise from situations such as the following:

(1) Some blood programs, especially those in which the recruiters are more comfortable working with the media than with individual organizations, may perform a considerable part of their routine recruitment by means of a crisis image in the mass media. (I know of one case where a reporter tried to document the "crisis" and came up with pretty embarrassing results.) The use of such messages for routine collections could well give the public reason to be unsure of its blood supply and skeptical of its blood collectors.

(2) The "premiums" in IR systems are often necessarily too high to be called premiums. Usually, the people whose blood needs are being insured are also providing for the blood needs of the larger community. It may be important that the donors be told this by the blood system before they learn it from other parties. As one example, consider a "stork club" arrangement, in which parents are asked to have donors predeposit several units of blood to cover possible blood needs at the time their child is delivered. A news story comparing this enormous "premium" with the likelihood of the need for transfusions when a baby is delivered would do little for the image of the blood-collection system. I do not object if the prospective parents are told that the stork club is simply a traditional means by which the community raises part of its blood supply. But any implication that the donations are justified in terms of likely needs associated with the birth seems to me to threaten the integrity of the entire system.

(3) Some programs which describe themselves as CR-SG use recruiting messages and materials that are not at all consistent with that ideology. Such messages often hint that some tentatively serious aspect of the treatment a patient

121

receives depends on whether that person has obtained "coverage." If the system is actually CR-SG, the message is not true and could cause public relations problems if exposed. If the message is true, the blood-collection system should simply describe itself as IR in accord with its practices. (Of course, this can be an especially difficult issue for systems trying to change ideologies.)

Coexistence between Different Ideologies. Although this issue is sometimes over-played in the relations between the major blood-collection organizations, it clearly is important to find some fair arrangement for coexistence between IR and CR systems. The ideological differences between these systems do not affect most aspects of blood use and, to my way of thinking, the problem of coexistence is something the major collectors could resolve if they were strongly motivated to do so. To me, it seems both preferable and easier to solve this problem than to attempt to impose a uniform blood-collection ideology on the entire country.

Summary

In this discussion paper, I have offered a framework for organizing blood-collection ideologies, and I have noted some of the reasons why practices are often more similar than ideologies. I have included a brief sample of my own research project. Then, moving beyond the level of knowledge available, I have presented my personal conjectures about the blood supply as it exists today and suggested some of the more important issues that concern it.

One of my conclusions is that the selection of a blood-collection ideology need not necessarily have a major effect on most of the important measures of blood-system performance. At the present level of needs, there appear to be many ways for a community to obtain its blood supply. It seems to me that too many people hope to "resolve" issues that are ideological by studying the per-formance of existing systems.

More generally, I see only very limited evidence that the blood-supply system lives up to the terrible publicity it often receives (and which it sometimes seems to foster and enjoy). I have indicated my own priorities for attention. I am very enthusiastic about the general directions suggested in the report of the ABC Task Force on Regional Association of Blood Service Units. I would be hesitant to force major changes upon blood-supply systems that already provide broad areas with excellent supplies in terms of adequacy, availability, efficiency, and purity. Interventions on ideological grounds should be described for what they are, rather than as attempts to improve these aspects of the supply.

It is clear that much of what I have said is subjective and interpretive. I hope my presentation can serve as one more basis for organizing and evaluating the major issues on the supply side of the blood-service system in the United States.

PERFORMANCE MEASURES FOR NONPROFIT BLOOD SYSTEMS

Edward L. Wallace

Until recently most nonprofit regional blood bankers were happily unaware of the concepts of effectiveness and efficiency and of the role these concepts ought to play in the conduct of regional blood-system operations. Regional blood banking, with a few notable exceptions, has been a closed affair conducted like a charitable activity on a best-efforts basis with minimum expenditure of financial resources. Efforts by the Department of Health, Education, and Welfare through the promulgation of the National Blood Policy and the organization of the American Blood Commission have begun to alter the situation. Blood has been assigned a prominent role in the ongoing debate over health policy, and the public responsibilities of blood bankers have been defined.

A major part of this HEW effort has been to stimulate the national blood community through the American Blood Commission to organize itself into a comprehensive system of blood regions with a national blood-data center to compile, analyze, and report information relevant to blood-system operations in the United States. A comprehensive regional system of blood operations is viewed by many as the keystone of a truly national blood system and the organizational imperative for improving the effectiveness and efficiency of present blood-service operations. The development of a comprehensive system of performance measures for regional blood systems will assist in identifying the magnitudes and sources of present ineffectiveness and inefficiency and, it is hoped, stimulate efforts to improve operations.

Requirements for Performance: Assessment and Operating Improvements

It is important to note that performance measures constitute only a part of the larger set of requirements of a system aimed at improving effectiveness and efficiency. Of even greater importance is the grouping of individual small blood-service establishments into regional organizations large enough to achieve economies of scale and with centralized authority and responsibility for regional planning and conduct of blood-service operations. Presumably, this is the purpose of the blood-service region that the American Blood Commission and its Task Force on Regionalization has in mind.

Given the existence of regional blood systems, it is necessary that they be organized with incentives to improve upon the present conduct of blood-service operations. In a nonprofit region this is usually best accomplished by the creation of a peer-review organization and a process to evaluate performance and to determine appropriate forms of administrative action to be carried out.

In order for a peer-review evaluation process to function effectively it is also necessary to establish a system of data collection and analysis and to develop a set of generally agreed-upon performance measures and standards appropriate to each.

In the United States the development of such a system of comprehensive regions served by well-designed information systems capable of assisting in the planning and control of operations is not a simple task. Forces certain to delay and possibly thwart the proposed development include the following: the present diffusion of authority and responsibility for blood-service operations among thousands of small quasi-independent blood-service establishments; the frequent lack of any real coordinating authority for blood-service operations in an area; the tradition of independence among small blood-service establishments, especially transfusion services and their national organization; the inertia and the disinclination to change that characterize many of the present regions; and a pervasive interest on investment minimization.

A further complication arises from the multidimensional character of the objectives of nonprofit blood operations. Since over 90 percent of all whole blood collected in the United States is collected by nonprofit organizations, the lack of a single clear objective—such as return on investment—as a comprehensive means for measuring the success of blood-service operations is an important difficulty. The goals of blood-service operations specified in the National Blood Policy, as will be seen, do not provide a solution to this problem, for these goals are too general to be operationally useful and lack criteria for choice in those situations where goal trade-offs are necessary.

The keys, then, to substantial improvement in the performance of blood-service operations in the United States appear to be (1) some degree of reorganization of blood-service establishments into regional groupings to permit the achievement of scale economies, (2) the centralization of authority for the planning and conduct of regional operations, (3) the development of peer-review processes for performance evaluation and administrative follow-up within regions, (4) development of regional information systems to assist in planning and in the conduct of the peer-review process, and (5) the development of performance measures that reflect the goals of regional blood-service operations and facilitate the planning and conduct of the performance-evaluation process.

The Goals and Subgoals of National Blood Policy. The first step in the development of a set of regional performance measures is specification of the goals of regional blood-service operations. The National Blood Policy defines four goals:

124

adequate supply, general accessibility, high quality, and efficiency. Of these, three—supply, accessibility, and efficiency—will be examined here, and means of measuring their achievement will be proposed. Quality, which refers largely to medical effectiveness, is the one goal that will not be discussed here since its measurement involves considerations distinctly different from those relevant to the other three.

All three goals are inadequately defined in the National Blood Policy to permit their direct use in the development of performance measures. Each is a complex of subgoals. The supply and accessibility goals, for example, appear to be divisible into four distinct subgoals. Whether or not either general goal has been achieved can best be determined by the extent to which the subgoals of each are accomplished. These subgoals, however, are not always consistent one with another, so that total goal accomplishment often can be assessed only by reference to the complex of performance measures that reflect subgoal accomplishments. In brief, there exists no single overall measure of performance of a regional blood system or of regional blood-system performance with respect to any single National Blood Policy goal.

Much the same is true of measures of regional efficiency, except that it is possible to measure overall efficiency in a financial sense through a single measure, provided the elements of that measure are available. Since financial efficiency is not usually considered the sole efficiency objective of regional actions, overall regional efficiency, like overall regional effectiveness, can be evaluated only indirectly through functional measures of efficiency. Thus, to be useful in the development of performance measures for regional blood systems, the general goals of National Blood Policy should be subdivided along the lines proposed below.

Adequacy of supply of blood products means that the region should provide:

(1) a *quantity* of each blood product required within a region sufficient to meet reasonable patient demand during the period,

(2) a *consistent* supply of each blood product in order to minimize outdating and shortages of blood products during the period,

(3) a *range* of blood products which reflects the variety of patient needs during the period, and

(4) a *mix* of blood products which reflects the relative quantities demanded by physicians on behalf of patients.

Similarly, the National Blood Policy goal of achieving accessibility to blood products for all persons within a region without regard to ability to pay can be subdivided into the subgoals of ensuring that:

125

(1) all patients and their physicians have whatever *information* is necessary to provide them knowledge of and access to the blood or plasma products most appropriate to their needs,

(2) all blood products be *distributed* within the region in a way which permits access to these products by those in need without unreasonable delays,

(3) the *price* or other method of charging for the use of each blood product does not preclude its usage in amounts that are medically desirable, and

(4) the *utilization* of all blood products within the region conforms to a usage pattern consistent with good medical practice.

These eight subgoals of supply and accessibility can be useful guides to regional action, directing it towards activities that will achieve the general goals of National Blood Policy.

Similarly, it is desirable to subdivide the efficiency goal. In this case, however, the subdivision does not reflect subgoals but rather, different methods of measuring output or input in the efficiency measure. Four types of efficiency measures are proposed:

(1) a *general* measure based on value of output and costs of input,

(2) a *cost* measure based on units of output and costs of input,

(3) a *man-hour* measure based on units of output and man-hours of input, and

(4) a *yield* measure based on units of output and units of input.

Each type of measure is useful under appropriate circumstances.

Functions of a Regional Blood System. The activities that typify a complete regional blood system involve eight separable but related functions. By examining each function it is possible to identify more precisely the subgoals of National Blood Policy that each function aims to achieve and the measures of effectiveness and efficiency relevant to it. All functions do not aim directly at the achievement of all National Blood Policy subgoals. Some functions aim at achieving subgoals which are necessary precursors of and means of achieving the national goals. Finally, performance measures for appropriate combinations of national subgoals and regional functions are not always possible and surrogate measures are necessary.

The functions of a regional blood system to be considered here are: (1) recruiting of donors, (2) collection of whole blood and plasma, (3) processing of whole blood and plasma, (4) distribution of blood products, (5) transfusion of blood products, (6) education of donors, patients, physicians, and others associated with the regional system, (7) research and consultation in blood-service

126

management methods, and (8) management of the regional system. The first four are the functions usually identified with regional operations and, together with the fifth function, which is normally performed by hospitals, constitute the process by which blood products are created, distributed, and used to meet patient needs. The last three functions are different. Each is distinct from the others and from the first five as a group. They represent other dimensions of regional action.

Proposed Measures of Effectiveness and Efficiency. In developing measures for evaluating the effectiveness of regional blood-system operations it is easiest to begin with each function to be evaluated and relate it to the subgoals it aims to achieve. Table 1 illustrates this approach by listing the eight principal functions and the twelve subgoals to be achieved, or methods of efficiency measurement to be used, in columns. Each row-column intersection, or cell, represents a possible goal-directed activity. Performance measures for each goal-directed activity are listed in Table 1 in the relevant cells by alphametric code (M1, M2, and so on), and selected key measures from the total set are described in Table 2. Since all regional functions do not attempt to achieve all subgoals or make use of all possible efficiency measures, many of the cells in Table 1 do not contain performance-measure references. Nonetheless, fifty-seven different possible measures have been defined for consideration.

Obviously it is not useful here to describe in detail each of the fifty-seven proposed measures. Instead attention will be given to thirteen of these that are believed to be most significant. This same approach is proposed for eventual use in evaluating regional operations in order to reduce to a manageable size the number of measures being reported and to concentrate attention on performance of the significant aspects of regional operations.

Donor recruiting. The purpose of donor recruiting is to create and maintain the pool of regional donors. An important consideration is the size of the active regional donor pool relative to the size of the eligible regional population. M1 measures this. It also indicates the kind of recruiting strategy being employed by the region, either emphasis on a small but efficient donor pool with frequent bleeding or emphasis on a large comprehensive pool emphasizing extensive community involvement. By combining M35 or M37, both of which are measures of recruiting efficiency, with M1 for different regions, it should be possible to gain insights into the relative efficiencies of the concentrated-donor-pool strategy as compared with the comprehensive-donor-pool strategy. This is important information that is lacking today.

Collections. Collections effectiveness is easier to assess than recruiting effectiveness. M5 provides the principal means of doing this by relating the physical quantity of blood or plasma collected to a proxy measure of potential supply, the eligible population of the region. The efficiency of collections can be estimated by

127

Table 1

RELATIONSHIP OF PROPOSED MEASURES OF EFFECTIVENESS AND EFFICIENCY TO THE FUNCTIONS OF A REGIONAL BLOOD SYSTEM AND THE GOALS OF NATIONAL BLOOD POLICY

(in alphametric code)

Regional Blood-System Functions	National Blood Policy Goals											
	Effectiveness								Efficiency			
	Supply				Accessibility				Types of measures			
	Quantity	Consistency	Range	Mix	Information	Distribution	Price	Utilization	General	Man-hours	Cost	Yield
1. Donor recruiting	M1	M2	M3 M4	M3 M4						M35 M36	M37 M38	M41
2. Collection	M5	M6 M7	M8 M9	M8 M9						M39	M40	
3. Processing												
4. Distribution	M10 M11	M13		M12		M14 M15 M16 M17	M18			M42 M44	M43 M45	M46 M47
5. Transfusion	M19 M20 M27	M22 M23		M21			M24 M25	M26				M48 M49
6. Education										M51	M50	
7. Research and consultation	M28 M29 M30 M31									M52 M53 M54	M55	
8. Management	M32 M33								M34	M56	M57	

Note: For example see text, p. 127. For a detailed breakdown of table entries see Table 2.
Source: Edward L. Wallace.

Table 2

PROPOSED MEASURES OF REGIONAL
BLOOD-SYSTEM EFFECTIVENESS AND EFFICIENCY

The performance measures proposed below are possible means of evaluating the effectiveness and efficiency of regional blood systems in attaining the supply, accessibility, and efficiency goals of National Blood Policy. Each measure is identified by a code number which refers to the particular combination of regional blood-system function and National Blood Policy subgoal achievement which the measure proposes to assess. These combinations of functions and subgoals to which each performance measure refers can be found in Table 1, where the code number of each measure is shown at the intersection of the function and the subgoal to which it corresponds.

MEASURES OF EFFECTIVENESS

Donor Recruiting

Quantity

$$M1 = \frac{\text{Number of individuals donating whole blood or plasma over the past years}}{\text{Total regional population age 17-64}}$$

Consistency

$$M2 = \frac{\text{Number of repeat donors used during the past year}}{\text{Total number of donors during past year}}$$

Range and Mix

$$M3 = \frac{\text{Number of special donors used during past 3 years}}{\text{Number of donors used during past 3 years}}$$

$$M4 = \frac{\text{Number of on-call donors used during past 3 years}}{\text{Number of donors used during past 3 years}}$$

Collections

Quantity

$$M5 = \frac{\text{Total units of whole blood and plasma collected during year}}{\text{Total regional population age 17-64}}$$

Consistency

$$M6 = \text{Average monthly deviation of collections of whole blood and plasma from mean monthly collections for the past year}$$

$$M7 = \frac{\text{Number of whole-blood, plasma, or blood-product units imported monthly by RBS}}{\text{Regional average monthly collections}}$$

Range and mix

$$M8 = \frac{\text{Number of special types of whole-blood or plasma units collected during year}}{\text{Total whole-blood or plasma units collected during year}}$$

$$M9 = \frac{\text{Number of special types of whole-blood or plasma units imported during year}}{\text{Total whole-blood or plasma units collected during year}}$$

Table 2 (continued)

MEASURES OF EFFECTIVENESS (continued)

Distribution

Quantity

$$M10 = \frac{\text{Number of blood-product units produced}}{\text{Total population of region}}$$

$$M11 = \frac{\text{Number of units of each blood product produced}}{\text{Total population of region}}$$

Consistency

M12 = Average deviation of monthly production of each blood product from mean monthly production

$$M13 = \frac{\text{Percent of total regional production going to each blood product produced by region}}{\text{Percent of average total production nationally going to each blood product}}$$

Distribution

$$M14 = \frac{\text{Average daily regional inventory of blood product}}{\text{Average daily regional transfusions}}$$

$$M15 = \frac{\text{Average daily regional inventory of each blood product}}{\text{Average daily regional transfusions of each blood product}}$$

$$M16 = \frac{\text{Average daily inventory in each hospital}}{\text{Average daily transfusions in each hospital}}$$

$$M17 = \frac{\text{Average daily size of hospital inventory by blood-product type}}{\text{Average daily transfusions of each blood product in each hospital}}$$

Price

$$M18 = \frac{\text{Prices of each regional blood product including replacement fees}}{\text{Average national price of each blood product including replacement fees}}$$

Transfusion

Quantity

$$M19 = \frac{\text{Units of blood products transfused during period}}{\text{Thousands of total regional population}}$$

$$M20 = \frac{\text{Units of each blood product transfused during period}}{\text{Thousands of total regional population}}$$

Consistency

M21 = Average deviation of units of blood products transfused monthly in region from mean monthly total units transfused

M22 = Average deviation of units of each blood product transfused monthly from mean monthly units of each blood product transfused

Range and Mix

$$M23 = \frac{\text{Units of each blood product transfused during year}}{\text{Units of all blood products transfused during year}}$$

Table 2 (continued)

MEASURES OF EFFECTIVENESS (continued)

Price

$$M24 = \frac{\text{Average price per blood-product unit transfused in the region}}{\text{Average national price per blood-product unit transfused}}$$

$$M25 = \frac{\text{Average price of each blood-product unit transfused in region}}{\text{National average price of each blood-product unit transfused}}$$

Utilization

$$M26 = \frac{\text{Percent of total units of each blood product transfused in the region}}{\text{Percent of total units of each blood product transfused nationally}}$$

Education

Quantity

$$M27 = \frac{\text{Total man-hours spent on regional education}}{\text{National average man-hours spent on education}}$$

Research and Consultation

Quantity

$$M28 = \frac{\text{Total man-hours spent on regional research}}{\text{Total man-hours spent in the region}}$$

$$M29 = \frac{\text{Total regional research man-hours}}{\text{National average of regional man-hours spent on research}}$$

$$M30 = \frac{\text{Number of regional consultations}}{\text{Total number of transfusions in the region}}$$

$$M31 = \frac{\text{Total regional man-hours spent on consultation}}{\text{National average of regional man-hours spent on consultation}}$$

Management

Quantity

$$M32 = \frac{\text{Man-hours of professional management in the region}}{\text{National average number of professional management man-hours per region}}$$

$$M33 = \frac{\text{Average annual compensation of professional management in the region}}{\text{National average annual compensation for professional management for all regions}}$$

MEASURES OF EFFICIENCY

Management

General

$$M34 = \frac{\text{Total value of all useful regional outputs of blood products and services}}{\text{Total cost of all regional operations}}$$

Donor Recruiting

Man-hours

$$M35 = \frac{\text{Number of donors donating during the past year}}{\text{Man-hours spent on donor recruiting in region}}$$

Table 2 (continued)

MEASURES OF EFFICIENCY (continued)

$$M36 = \frac{\text{Number of new donors donating during past year}}{\text{Man-hours spent on donor recruiting in region}}$$

Costs

$$M37 = \frac{\text{Number of donors donating during period}}{\text{Total cost of regional recruiting during period}}$$

$$M38 = \frac{\text{Number of new donors donating during period}}{\text{Total cost of regional recruiting during period}}$$

Collection
Man-hours

$$M39 = \frac{\text{Whole-blood and plasma units collected}}{\text{Total man-hours spent on collection}}$$

Costs

$$M40 = \frac{\text{Whole-blood and plasma units collected}}{\text{Total costs of collection}}$$

Processing
Yield

$$M41 = \frac{\text{Total number of blood-product units produced}}{\text{Total number of whole-blood and plasma units collected}}$$

Man-hours

$$M42 = \frac{\text{Total number of blood-product units produced}}{\text{Total man-hours used in processing}}$$

Cost

$$M43 = \frac{\text{Total number of blood-product units produced}}{\text{Total cost of processing}}$$

Distribution
Man-hours

$$M44 = \frac{\text{Total number of blood-product units distributed}}{\text{Total man-hours spent on distribution}}$$

Cost

$$M45 = \frac{\text{Total number of blood-product units distributed}}{\text{Total cost of distribution}}$$

Yield

$$M46 = \frac{\text{Average daily inventory of blood products}}{\text{Average daily production of blood products}}$$

$$M47 = \frac{\text{Total blood-product units not transfused}}{\text{Total blood-product units produced}}$$

Table 2 (continued)

MEASURES OF EFFICIENCY (continued)

Transfusion

Yield

$$M48 = \frac{\text{Total blood-product units transfused}}{\text{Total whole-blood and plasma units collected}}$$

$$M49 = \frac{\text{Total blood-product units transfused}}{\text{Total blood-product units produced}}$$

Education

Cost

$$M50 = \frac{\text{Total numbers of technicians, physicians, staff members, or promotional messages sent}}{\text{Cost of education of technicians, physicians, and staff members or of promotional messages sent}}$$

Man-hours

$$M51 = \frac{\text{Regional man-hours expended on various types of education}}{\text{Whole-blood and plasma units collected}}$$

Research and Consultation

Man-hours

$$M52 = \frac{\text{Research or consultation man-hours}}{\text{Blood-product units produced}}$$

$$M53 = \frac{\text{Research or consultation man-hours}}{\text{Whole-blood and plasma units collected}}$$

Cost

$$M54 = \frac{\text{Number of consultation man-hours}}{\text{Number of consultations}}$$

$$M55 = \frac{\text{Cost of consultations}}{\text{Number of consultations}}$$

Management

Man-hours

$$M56 = \frac{\text{Man-hours of professional management}}{\text{Total number of whole-blood and plasma units collected}}$$

Cost

$$M57 = \frac{\text{Cost of regional management}}{\text{Total number of whole-blood and plasma units collected}}$$

Source: Edward L. Wallace.

M39 or M40. In combination, M5 and M39 or M40 can provide useful insights into the relative efficiencies of different possible collections strategies, thereby providing knowledge of potential benefits and costs of different collections methods.

133

Processing. Processing is an intermediate function of great importance to the overall operating efficiency of regional operations. Knowledge of the yield of blood products from processing, as reflected in M41, or processing costs, as reflected by M43, provides information vital to the resolution of such policy-related questions as what are the extent and sources of economies of scale in regional blood operations or what economies may be achieved by extending the range and mix of blood products produced regionally. These are issues about which little is now known.

Distribution. Distributive effectiveness is measurable in several different ways. One measure of considerable importance is M14, which reflects the ratio of the average regional daily supply of blood products to average daily use. Too high a supply relative to use means a substantial risk of overstocking and loss from outdating; too low a supply relative to use means a substantial risk of under-stocking and shortages. What we would like to know is what constitute effective and efficient regional collections and inventory strategies for regions with different operating characteristics. Today we really do not know what these might be, but with performance measures such as M14 and additional data on various regional characteristics it will be possible to identify and evaluate these strategies.

Transfusion. Transfusion differs from distribution in that it refers to actual use of blood products as distinct from their mere availability. Three aspects of regional transfusion activity are of special importance. First, there is the quantity of each blood product transfused each period in relationship to the region's population. This relationship is measured by M20 and is one useful indicator of the medical effectiveness of a region's blood program.

Second, the price of transfused products is an important indicator of both the accessibility of the region's blood products and the region's financial efficiency. M25 provides a measure of both aspects of regional operations since it relates the regional prices of blood products to national prices.

The third important aspect of regional transfusion activity is the efficiency of transfusion yield as measured by M48. This measure has long been used in blood banking as an indicator of operating efficiency, perhaps too much so, for it measures the regional average rate of blood-product outdating. We know from past studies that blood-product outdating is high in the United States; what we do not know is why. By relating regional experiences on M48 to other regional characteristics it should be possible to identify the main causes of unusually high outdating and, possibly, to develop effective forms of corrective action.

Other regional functions. Similar measures are possible for other regional functions: education, research and consultation, and management. Of principal interest to the management function is M34, the measure which relates total value of useful regional outputs to total regional cost. This comprehensive revenue-cost ratio shows the financial viability of the region, a matter of considerable concern especially when it is coupled with comparative price information such as that proposed in M25.

Implementation Experience. Developing a system of performance measures for a regional blood system is one matter; implementing it in ways which will alter the incentives and behavior patterns of regional personnel is another. As previously indicated, there are a number of other requirements to be developed in concert with a system of regional performance measures before improvements in effectiveness and efficiency are likely: establishment or restructuring of the regional organization, creation of a peer review procedure and standards of performance, development of the necessary supportive information systems, and establishment of an administrative follow-up and reporting process. Without these the total management system will be lacking essential elements and will be likely to fail.

Our limited experience with regional performance measures that we have developed and implemented in a medium-sized blood region bears this out. We produced for the region a series of measures that indicated such important information as the following: outdating of blood products was averaging over 25 percent; many individual blood establishments were carrying quantities of inventory that were, in some instances, three times the expected demand, with less than a one-in-twenty chance of creating shortages; the average age of blood products transfused was very high and thus their medical effectiveness reduced; and far too few packed red cells and other blood components were being transfused.

The result of having available this kind of regional performance information was most interesting. It obviously was a source of embarrassment to all. Since no peer review procedures existed, performance evaluation was the responsibility of the regional staff. The staff made a few half-hearted attempts to act on the information by discussing it with some of the affiliated blood establishments. This effort was largely unsuccessful because both the regional staff and the staffs of the individual blood establishments were not convinced that improving affiliated blood-establishment performances was the region's responsibility. In addition both recognized that the region lacked performance standards and a peer review process that could provide guidance and the authority to induce compliance with standards. So what was done was to eliminate the problem not by resolving it but rather by shifting the information system to a new computer and in the process eliminating the performance-measurement system. The point is, while effectiveness and efficiency may be needed in regional blood systems and performance measures can point the way to this end, performance measures alone are not enough. As long as the other necessary components of a total management system are lacking, performance measures will be nothing but an embarrassment to be ignored if they cannot be eliminated.

THE NEED FOR REFORM

Aaron Kellner

I should start with an apology. I confess that I had never heard of Reuben Kessel before the planning of this meeting. Since this meeting was dedicated to him, I obtained a copy of his paper "Transfused Blood, Serum Hepatitis, and the Coase Theorem" [see Appendix B]. I must apologize also to Professor Coase. I originally thought Coase—presumably a new enzyme—must be pronounced "Ko-ace." I read the paper carefully and was enormously impressed. It is beautifully written, tightly reasoned, and very scholarly. Then it dawned on me that there are many people out there who are wise, thoughtful, and scholarly, who are thinking about our problems, who have things to say to which we ought to be listening even if we disagree, but about whom I, and I am sure many of my colleagues, have never heard. This was an eye-opener for me. And so, in thanking the American Enterprise Institute and David Johnson, I should express the hope that this conference will not be the last of such interactions. I, for one, and I think other blood bankers too, would find them very salutary.

I have had the good fortune to see blood-banking systems in many different parts of the world. When one compares them objectively and critically, the pluralistic system we have developed in this country stacks up very well. It has collected large amounts of blood and plasma; it has effectively met most, if not all, the clinical needs of patients; and, more than any other system, it has been innovative and responsive to medical and technical advances. However, it has not been perfect.

The Weaknesses of Our Blood System

For purposes of this afternoon's presentation, since this is a program sponsored by AEI's Center for Health Policy Research and in view of the subject assigned to me, I have chosen six or seven nontechnical, nonhematological problem areas, soft spots that I see in the system, where we as operating blood bankers have, in our own fumbling way, tried to evolve social policy. I would warn you in advance— and with some trepidation—that all of these areas are quite controversial.

Responsibility. The first of these, and the single most important problem facing us, as I see it, is an ideological one, the question of who is to be responsible for

137

the blood supply. I do not agree with my friend and colleague, Alvin Drake, that it is not an important question. It is a key issue and the root cause of most of the unpleasant and passionate public controversy to which we have subjected ourselves.

Who is to be responsible for the blood supply, the community or the individual, the healthy or the sick? We have heard much about that already today. It is true that in actual operational form these alternative positions become fuzzy, but in their pure forms they are dramatically opposed. One group says, the community as a whole accepts responsibility for all blood needs. We give blood because our town, region, or country needs it. The other, espousing the idea of individual responsibility, says that people who have received blood should replace it. When we get something, we have an obligation to return it. In my view, the latter position, the idea of individual responsibility, leads inevitably to a cumbersome and now archaic superstructure of credits and debits, replacement and nonreplacement fees, blood assurance, the clearinghouse, and all the rest. I will not go into all these but will touch on one or two. Blood assurance is semantically misleading. The one thing it does not do is assure blood. What it does do is guarantee a discount if a donor should need blood later on. The donor gets transfusions at a lower cost. The nonreplacement fee, again, is a financial mechanism and, in my view, a punitive financial mechanism. A person who has not given blood must pay a surcharge. One group obtains a bargain, the other group is subjected to what some people have called a financial "ripoff."

In the discussion of these issues among blood bankers—and they are discussed, sometimes quite acrimoniously—two positions are often expressed. One is that the nonreplacement fee is an absolutely essential recruitment tool, that a blood supply cannot be obtained without it. That is clearly not true. The converse, however, is true; those who advocate individual responsibility and the nonreplacement fee operate successful blood programs. On the other hand, it is possible to operate a fully successful blood program without the club of the nonreplacement fee and without placing the onus of soliciting blood on the sick precisely at the time when they are least able to bear the burden of an additional responsibility. Communities can satisfy their blood needs without this cruel bludgeon; there is abundant evidence for this, both in this country and abroad.

There is another group which wants both systems to coexist, with freedom of choice between them—the position Dr. Drake mentioned a few minutes ago. This would be possible if each region in this country were a watertight compartment, without any interaction with other regions, but we do not operate that way. The population is a mobile one; people travel great distances for specialized health care, and at the regional interfaces between the two different philosophies friction and conflict inevitably would develop. I am reluctantly compelled to conclude that the two systems are essentially incompatible in any one region or in the country. I think the struggle will be fierce and the trauma great, but the outcome is inevitable. The concept of community responsibility will, in time, win out. The entire Red Cross system, which represents by itself 40 percent of America's blood supply, has, as you know, recently opted out of the clearinghouse and will shortly move to total community coverage, as will major non-Red Cross regional centers: the blood services of Arizona, Milwaukee, Seattle, Pittsburgh, New York, and many other places. The defenders of individual responsibility will be a minority fighting a valiant rear-guard action; but they will lose. I wish there were some compatible middle ground, and I hope Al Drake will turn out to be correct in his assertion that coexistence is possible, but I do not see any evidence that it is.

Voluntarism

The second big issue is that of voluntarism and about that we have heard a good deal today. The recent Bureau of Biologics proposal for labeling blood as paid or volunteer has created a highly inflammatory confrontation, and my guess is that within a year we will have a regulation for labeling blood and a definition—some simple operating definition, probably the transfer of dollars—by which we can determine whether blood is paid or voluntary.

Labeling is not really the issue, however. Even with labeling and with a definition, we have only scratched the surface. The real question is, Why do we want a voluntary blood supply? Is it to reduce the prevalence of hepatitis as outlined in the Bureau of Biologics' *Federal Register* statement or for broader social or moral reasons?

Professor Paul Samuelson, in his review of the Titmuss book, said that blood is much like love; the kind you get for free is better than the kind you get for money. Would those who think that blood should be voluntarily donated because donated blood is safer still prefer an all-volunteer system if there were a perfect test for hepatitis?

This morning one could easily have acquired the impression that altruism was an undesirable thing, that it was something to be ashamed of, something shady, and that it was wrong to be emotional about anything. There is a strong feeling in this country—and I tend to share it—that the reason we want a voluntary blood supply is that altruism is a good thing, and we ought to be proud of it. In an acquisitive society, we ought to make every effort to maximize opportunities for altruism; we ought to create situations in which people care for each other, opportunities for giving and caring and sharing. As Dr. Gill, chairman of ABC's task force on donor recruitment, said to his task force yesterday, "Nothing is more symbolic of the relationship between one man and another than sharing blood."

Even with the perfect test for hepatitis, we would still want a voluntary blood supply, because a society that has a totally voluntary and altruistic blood supply is a better society. Despite Watergate, America is a highly moral society, and it will wish to remove all human tissues—hearts, kidneys, blood, and plasma—from the commercial marketplace.

There are other questions that need to be raised in connection with voluntarism. One of these is the question of plasma. Plasma presents a very difficult question that we must face. Dr. Meyer touched on it in his talk, but the rest of us have carefully skirted it; we have swept it under the rug. Can we tolerate the gross inconsistency of a totally volunteer blood supply side by side with a plasma supply that comes almost entirely from prisoners and paid donors? We have, in this country, been collecting fantastically large amounts of plasma, 3 million liters or more of plasma a year, and exploiting human beings as plasma protein factories.

Now, if we feel that this is wrong, how are we going to get enough plasma to provide the albumin, the immune globulins, the factor VIII, and the very important therapeutic modalities that we make out of plasma? It would not be easy.

Someone this morning talked about voluntary plasmapheresis, which we have hardly tried at all in this country. It is being tried in England. I was in Belgium a couple of weeks ago and the Belgium Red Cross runs, with very little effort, a beautiful voluntary plasmapheresis program which yields 10,000 liters of plasma a year—a small amount by our standards, but Belgium is a small country. I was quite surprised to find that housewives, school teachers, students, storekeepers come in once or twice a month for a voluntary double plasmapheresis. A similar program, successfully operated, is underway in Finland. In Milwaukee, in this country, they have been able to get volunteers for plateletpheresis. We cannot dodge the issue indefinitely; we are going to have to face it. We have allowed the pharmaceutical industry to develop social policy for us. Or, perhaps even worse, we have developed social policy by default. The question of plasma is a very difficult one, but we have to look into it if we are honest about a totally volunteer blood supply.

Data and Disclosure. A third soft spot is the matter of statistics. It is ironic indeed that a country that can put men on the moon almost at will, that knows with a high degree of precision how much water is flowing in the Mississippi River and how many potatoes were planted in Idaho, does not know how much blood is collected each year or what happens to it.

The only year in history for which we have reasonably reliable figures is 1971, when the management consulting firm Booz, Allen & Hamilton conducted a national survey for the National Institutes of Health. Even in that study, 29 percent of the blood was labeled unaccounted for, outdated, or otherwise lost, strayed, or stolen. Except for that year, we have only guesses and approximations. The situation is spotty. The state of New Jersey, for example, does a very good job. New York State does a miserable job. The Red Cross does a very good job on national statistics, the Council of Community Blood Centers does a middling to poor job, and the American Association of Blood Banks does no better.

Reliable data are essential for a system that expects to plan rationally, to know what is going on, to assess trends and to monitor performance. If we do not monitor our performance, the government will do it for us. That is why some of us have strongly advocated development of a national blood-data center and urged the creation of an American Blood Commission task force to accomplish that end. A national blood-data center would be the cornerstone for the implementation of the National Blood Policy. It is hard to see how the policy could be implemented without it. The Task Force on Regionalization of the American Blood Commission has recently recommended the creation of such a national blood-data center. The report was accepted and approved, though not without some dissent, at the last meeting of the board of directors of ABC. It looks as if we will, at long last, have a data center as a collaborative enterprise between ABC, the Bureau of Biologics, and the National Heart, Lung, and Blood Institute.

While on the subject of statistics, I should say a word about another, not generally appreciated, sore point—at least a sore point with me—and that is disclosure. Blood centers have the responsibility of disclosing fully to the public not only what they do with the blood they collect but also what they do with the dollars they collect. We cannot, in all honesty, expect people to give you their blood voluntarily and then hide from them how you spend their dollars. Blood centers are public corporations, and they should level with the public; there should be no secrets. There are a few blood centers that publish detailed or summary financial statements. However, detailed public disclosure, particularly of fiscal information has, unfortunately, been the exception rather than the rule. The point is easily proved by writing to the ten largest regional blood centers to ask for annual reports for the last five years.

Concern for the Patient. My fifth point deals with concern for the patient, a shibboleth loudly espoused by all blood-bank groups. It has, in critical situations, been more a slogan than a reality.

Let me cite a couple of instances because time is running short. When the Medicare regulations were being developed some ten years ago, the blood-bank community lobbied vigorously and effectively to exclude the first three units of blood or packed cells from coverage. We won the right to demand replacement for the first three pints of blood or to exact a replacement fee. This, mind you, from sick people, past the age of sixty-five, many of whom are alone and far from their children. This, in retrospect, was a needless and callous affront to the elderly. The Social Security Administration has ruled that nonprofit regional blood centers may, at their option, replace blood for Medicare patients, so that Medicare patients can be completely covered and would not be expected to pay a responsibility fee even for the first three units of blood. I wonder how many regional blood centers have taken advantage of this opportunity.

141

Another instance—and this has been cited frequently this morning—in recent years, blood banks and hospitals, concerned about the devastating possibilities of suits for hepatitis under the doctrine of implied warranty of product liability, rushed to their state legislatures to have blood made a service rather than a commodity. This was understandable, for even without negligence on their part and even when they had taken all possible precautions, there was still the risk of transmitting hepatitis, and they legitimately sought protection.

They were successful in most cases, and, by a bit of legal alchemy, blood became a service. Everybody was home free, everybody that is, except the innocent victim, the patient. After all, the patient who contracts hepatitis from a transfusion is blameless, too. Without fault on his part and as an unexpected and unpreventable complication of his treatment, he is subjected to prolonged hospitalization, loss of income, and even death. Yet, no one gave a thought to his hurt; not the Red Cross, not the AABB, not even the New York Blood Center. In our zeal for exculpation, we never thought of helping the patient.

There are social mechanisms such as worker's compensation to help the working man who is injured on the job; there are attempts to compensate the innocent victims of crime and national disaster; and we heard a good deal this morning about no-fault insurance. Yet in the medical and blood-banking community, to the best of my knowledge, not a voice was raised in defense of the victim of post-transfusion hepatitis. We could at least have pointed out the inequity, but we did not. We were concerned with our own peril; where was our concern for the patient? Our so-called concern for the patient is really superficial and self-serving. We need to rethink our position and reexamine the level of our social consciousness.

Governance and Regionalization. The next point I will touch on, briefly, is a matter of some concern; it is the governance of regional blood centers. The policy-making body, the directors, the trustees, those who have broad public and fiscal responsibility for a regional blood center, should be representative of the community served, both lay and professional. Yet, if one looks about the country, one finds regional blood centers—large, respected, old regional blood centers—whose boards are dominated by doctors or composed exclusively of doctors. Some are even owned by medical societies. If it is unethical for a doctor to own a pharmacy, is it ethical for doctors to own a blood center? Some of us take a dim view of doctors owning a hospital; should we not take a similar view of doctors owning or dominating the board of a blood center? The matter of governance is not trivial. Governance is extremely important in the development of social policy. In fact, the domination of the boards of regional blood centers by physicians may, in part at least, be responsible for some of the mistakes we have made in the development of social policy. Doctors should not, by themselves, make social policy or health policy. They should have an important voice in the development of such policy, but in concert with others. This has not always been the case in the field of blood transfusion.

The last point I will make about America's blood service complex is its remarkable degree of fragmentation. Dr. Wallace and others have dwelt upon that at some length. There are over 5,000 separate blood-collection agencies in the United States. This is too large a number for efficient operation, for efficient allocation of sharing of resources, or even, for example, for the effective conservation of plasma. We need to look carefully at this heterogeneous mass of separate operating units and devise a way to phase out those that are operationally and hematologically inefficient and tie the remainder together into logical and workable networks. That is what regionalization is all about.

The case for regionalization has been very well expressed in the recently circulated report of ABC's task force on regionalization.[1] Many of you have seen it and some of you have even read it. I do not necessarily agree with every word, and particularly not with the section on implementation. It is, nevertheless, a splendid and highly commendable piece of work, though, of necessity, a compromise between conflicting points of view. It is a thoughtful, forward-looking, carefully written, and highly responsible document. It is easily the best analysis of blood-bank regionalization that I have ever seen. That is why I have been so surprised, really amazed, at the level of the critiques of the report that have been circulated recently. I urge you to read the report carefully and with an open mind. Read it not as Holy Writ, but as the first draft of a long-range plan; as a blueprint for the future that is intended to be examined, modified, and improved. It represents a significant step forward. I am convinced that most of the things outlined therein will come to pass.

A couple of points made in the report should be underscored. The purpose of regionalization is not to destroy small blood centers nor to create bigness for the sake of bigness. Its purpose is, where appropriate, to regroup and coordinate existing facilities so that they can render better service and make optimal use of available resources. This goal will require more than the creation of regional centers. It will require the creation of a new framework within which the regional centers and the hospital transfusion services can interact in sharing responsibility for patient care.

Two experiments in the creation of a new kind of association are being conducted in the Puget Sound area and in New York and Long Island, the latter known as LIBRA (Long Island Blood Resources Association), which is still in its formative stages. Our blood-collection facility on Long Island, which collects more than 120,000 units of blood a year, provides essentially all of the blood and blood services used in that encapsulated area. We are forming, together with the

---

[1] *Report of the Task Force on Regional Association of Blood Service Units* (Arlington, Virginia: American Blood Commission, July 15, 1976).

thirty-two hospitals we serve, a voluntary association with a policy-making board of directors consisting of representation from the hospitals, from other health agencies, and from the lay public. Instead of encouraging an adversary situation, a polarization between the regional blood centers and the hospitals they serve, we are trying to create a situation where the two will interact constructively. Together they are responsible for patient care.

Within LIBRA most of the quantitative functions that Dr. Wallace mentioned will be worked out by the regional center and the hospitals together—inspection and accreditation, for example. We have kept the Bureau of Biologics informed of our progress and expect in due course to apply for one of the regional licenses that Dr. Meyer mentioned in his address. Such things as blood collection and distribution, inventory management, quality control, performance testing, education, error tracking, record keeping, all the aspects of the relationship between regional blood centers and hospitals, will be worked out in concert. We hope that there will evolve a new collaborative relationship between the two to replace the present unsatisfactory purveyor-customer relationship.

COMMENTARIES

Ian Mitchell

I do not disagree with Professor Havighurst's remarks about the medical community. As a physician (though involved with organized medicine only through my position at HEW), I am deeply concerned about the fact that organized medicine does not always represent the interests of its own members or even the attitudes of its own members and that it does not always represent the needs of the people to be served.

I would like to run quickly through some salient points that occurred to me as I listened to the papers in the morning and afternoon sessions and then move on to some unfinished business from the morning session. First, the history of the development of the National Blood Policy should be clarified because Professor Havighurst suggested that the Department of Health, Education, and Welfare had gratuitously taken up this subject. HEW was not the first to call for action. There had been paper after paper in the scientific literature and in the blood-banking literature that said something needed to be done. There were developments in the private sector that cried out for attention from HEW, and HEW has a specific mandate to protect human health and welfare. When it proposed a policy, which is nothing more than a declaration of intent, it was only responding to that mandate. To suggest that somehow this policy was created by two or three people in the department and was not subjected to any kind of critical analysis is wholly misleading.

The policy itself was developed carefully within HEW over the period of a year. It was approved at the level of the secretary and then submitted to the Office of Management and Budget, where it was subjected to further review by other organizations in the government including the Department of Justice and the Department of Commerce. Before it was promulgated, it was discussed with the staffs of the various congressional health committees. They said generally that they thought it would accomplish little, that, if anything, it was too weak. However, they were willing to give it a try by tacitly agreeing not to interfere. We have tried very hard not to act gratuitously. We have tried very hard to obey what we believe to be our mandate.

I am surprised by the suggestion that the private sector, left to its own devices, would have done just as much and perhaps more. We have more than enough evidence that the private sector, when allowed to do its own thing, often serves its own ends first.

Let me cite a case in point; it occurred outside the United States, so no one in the United States need take umbrage. In the province of Ontario a bill was recently introduced into the legislature to penalize physicians involved with kickbacks in the ordering of or the performance of clinical lab tests. The simple introduction of that bill reportedly had the effect of decreasing the number of orders for clinical lab tests in various geographic areas by from 30 to 70 percent. That tells us something.

Comparing a blood transfusion to a dangerous occupation is dubious, to say the least. The person who chooses to work in a dangerous situation or to live in some dangerous way makes his own decision. The person who receives a transfusion, however, usually has no role in the decision. The recipient generally has no choice whether he will receive blood, nor does he decide upon the source of the blood or its quality. Let us not go on with the foolish pretense that blood is like all or any other consumer goods.

There has been the suggestion that HEW is about to impose central control, planning, and management. This is absolutely incorrect; in fact, the department insisted that the private sector be called upon to implement National Blood Policy. If anything, we are criticized for not imposing enough central control. We wanted to avoid going so far as to preempt the opportunity of the private sector to be creative.

Turning to unfinished business, I think people have tended to speculate and to philosophize on the basis of very little information and have failed to carry their speculation to its logical consequences. I have in mind Professor Kessel's paper[1] and the statement by the Council on Wage and Price Stability (COWPS).

On January 13, 1976, the staff of the Council on Wage and Price Stability issued and publicized a statement responding to the notice of proposed rule making published by the Food and Drug Administration on November 13, 1975. The proposed rule would require the labeling of blood as to source (volunteer donor or paid donor) and the addition of a warning on units obtained from paid donors.

In issuing its statement, the staff of the Council on Wage and Price Stability cited the authorities granted the council by the Congress in the Council on Wage and Price Stability Act of 1974.[2]

The chairman of the council stated: "The COWPS filing largely follows the analysis and recommendations of Professor Reuben Kessel as presented in his article, 'Transfused Blood, Serum Hepatitis, and the Coase Theorem,' "[3] about which much has been said today. Unfortunately, neither the late Professor Kessel

---

[1] Reuben Kessel, "Transfused Blood, Serum Hepatitis, and the Coase Theorem," *Journal of Law and Economics* (October 1974), pp. 265-89.

[2] Public Law 93-387, as amended by Public Law 94-78, 12 U.S.C. 1904 note.

[3] Letter to Dr. J. Garrott Allen from the chairman of the council, February 10, 1976.

nor the staff of the council actually provided an estimate of the cost of adopting the professor's proposal. It is therefore necessary to examine carefully what it was that Professor Kessel proposed before exploring its costs and implications.

Professor Kessel's proposal depends critically upon two concepts: first, that the blood-services community, broadly speaking, be held responsible for all injuries resulting from blood transfusions, whether or not negligence or fault was involved; and second, that a means be found of purging the donor population of all infectious donors.

Professor Kessel believed that the treatment of blood transfusions as products rather than services would bring into play the concept of implied warranty and the principle of strict liability in tort. He would have used the threat of financial injury, coupled with motivation by profit in a commercial setting, to compel the blood-services community to perform optimally; indeed to perform things it cannot yet do.

In addition to applying the best technology for the identification of infectious units of blood and employing monetary incentives to attract those donors who are regarded as the safest in respect to the quality of blood, there is only one means, conceptually, of purging the donor population of infectious donors: namely, a donor-recipient link. The donor-recipient link would, if successful, identify all donor sources in each case of hepatitis so that the infectious donor could be excluded from future donations.

There are several problems associated with the two concepts on which Professor Kessel's proposal rests. First, if the courts are persuaded to treat blood transfusions as products rather than services, the blood-services community probably will become liable for every kind of injury associated with blood transfusions, even in situations where nothing more could have been done to prevent the injuries. As will be shown later, this would be a highly dangerous development and certainly would risk increasing the cost of blood and blood services enormously.

The concept of the donor-recipient link was considered by the department's Task Force on Blood Banking, which concluded that it was both impracticable and exorbitantly expensive to implement except perhaps in narrowly defined situations. It relies upon follow-up of blood recipients, with extensive examination and testing for periods ranging up to six months. Follow-up of patients is frequently difficult and unreliable. If the patient is to be persuaded to go to expense and trouble there usually has to be some obvious potential benefit to the patient and, in the case of searching for transfusion-related hepatitis, there may be difficulty in persuading the individual that frequent reexamination is in his or her interest. This is particularly so where the patient's permanent residence is geographically distant from the site at which the follow-up examinations must occur. In addition, where the treating facility must rely upon other medical facilities to conduct the follow-up, consideration should be given to the interest and ability of the personnel with respect to searching for transfusion-related hepatitis. Finally, physicians burdened with paper work and possibly concerned about the legal consequences of reporting adverse effects of treatment may be disinclined to report the occurrence of transfusion-related hepatitis.

It would be difficult to persuade most patients that such follow-up is in fact in their interest, inasmuch as 95 percent of patients do not experience a lasting adverse effect from transfusions. Furthermore, the cost of the follow-up would have to be borne by someone; if not the patient directly, then the blood recipient, through charges for the blood services. Tracking down the donor population would be relatively easy and would not present a problem of great magnitude. However, where the recipient has been transfused from multiple donors, the problem of identifying the infectious donor(s) might be overwhelming.

If, as suggested by Professor Kessel, the blood-services community were to rely upon the smallest possible population of donors consistent with the demand for blood, it would be imperative that every infectious donor be identified. This would require following the medical courses of all recipients of blood, now more than 2.5 million patients per year. In this situation, where the opportunities to identify both overt and asymptomatic cases of hepatitis would be maximized, yet the correct identification of the responsible infectious source would be far from perfect, there must continue to be a substantial amount of hepatitis that was recognized but not preventable. This would maximize the exposure of the blood-services community to litigation under the concept of implied product warranty or strict liability in tort.

I have estimated the cost of a donor-recipient link at approximately $600 million per year. Two other people have estimated it as something more than twice that amount.[4] The cost of litigation, at least initially, would be about $560 million (16,000 $\times$ $35,000).[5] The incremental costs of donor incentives related to payments to attract the most appropriate donor population ($25.00 $-$ $7.50 $=$ $17.50)[6] would amount to $147 million per year. The total cost of implementing the Kessel proposal in the first year would be not less than $1.3 billion ($600 million $+$ $560 million $+$ $147 million $=$ $1.3 billion). It should be noted that this figure does not include the costs of litigation of cases of asymptomatic

---

[4] Memorandum from Dr. Lewellys F. Barker, director, Division of Blood and Blood Products, Food and Drug Administration, March 7, 1977; and letter from Dr. V. Paul Holland, chief, Blood Bank Department, Clinical Center, National Institutes of Health, March 8, 1977.

[5] Kessel's estimate of $23,225 as the cost of a case of symptomatic transfusion-related hepatitis in 1974, plus attorneys' fees of 30 percent, plus an inflationary factor of 7.5 percent per year not compounded. If the rate of symptomatic hepatitis resulting from transfusion of blood from a donor population which is 90 percent volunteer and 10 percent paid donors is 2.68, one would expect a total of 21,440 cases of symptomatic hepatitis. Employing the same assumptions but a rate of 2.0 cases of symptomatic hepatitis per 1,000 units transfused, as from an all-volunteer donor source, one would expect a total of 16,000 cases of symptomatic hepatitis.

[6] $7.50 approximates the payment to the commercial donor; $25.00 approximates the fee that noncommercial blood banks pay to their paid donors.

hepatitis, which under this system would be discovered more frequently than they are now and for which the injured party could then reasonably make a claim against the blood-services community. This situation would prevail because there are unquestionably cases of asymptomatic hepatitis that are discoverable only by chemical tests yet which result in chronic active hepatitis and progressive liver injury.

It is not possible at this point to project the full impact of the Kessel proposal from the medical or the economic viewpoint. But clearly its implementation would amount to an experiment of very large dimensions and risks, making the situation very much worse in terms of both health and economics, at least in the near future.

It is important to appreciate that the goal proposed by Kessel (two cases of symptomatic hepatitis per 1,000 units of blood transfused) is identical to that which both Grady and Kessel attributed to the current performance of the Red Cross and other volunteer donor groups.[7] It is also identical to Kessel's "best-quality blood supply."

An all-volunteer donor source, as distinguished from the current combination of paid and volunteer sources, would be expected to reach Kessel's goal without great experimentation or uncertainty. It would also do so without the enormous expense of the donor-recipient link.

While not agreeing entirely with the data and assumptions contained in the Grady and Kessel papers, I believe it appropriate in evaluating the Kessel paper and the council's statement (which is based on the Kessel paper) to accept, for these purposes only, those data. Kessel calculated that the average cost of a case of symptomatic transfusion-related hepatitis was $23,225 in 1974. He concluded that it would be worth $156 per unit of blood transfused to move from the poorest-quality blood to the best quality. On the basis of these figures and the assumption that current usage is 8 million units per year (that figure may be too low), Professor Kessel would have concluded that it was *worth* $1.25 billion per year to achieve his goal of two cases of symptomatic hepatitis per 1,000 units of blood transfused. But this can be done by adopting an all-volunteer supply without the expenditure of additional sums, much less the expenditure of $1.25 to $1.31 billion.

There is yet another way of examining the cost and worth of Kessel's proposal. The achievement of the goal of two cases per 1,000 units transfused would result in the prevention of approximately 5,540 cases[8] of symptomatic hepatitis per year, if one assumes Grady's data are correct. If the cost is divided by the

---

[7] George F. Grady, Ann J.E. Bennett et al., "Risk of Posttransfusion Hepatitis in the United States," *Journal of the American Medical Association*, vol. 220 (May 1, 1972), pp. 692-701.

[8] Assume that (a) Grady's data (footnote 7), (b) no recipient of a contaminated unit of blood receives more than one contaminated unit of blood, and (c) 8 million units of blood are transfused annually. A shift from a 90/10 mix of volunteer-to-paid donor population to an all-volunteer supply of blood would prevent approximately 5,540 (21,540 − 16,000 = 5,540) (see footnote 5) cases of symptomatic hepatitis per year.

benefit—that is, $1.31 billion divided by 5,540—the cost per case prevented is about $236,000 or approximately 10.2 times what Kessel estimated was the cost of a case of symptomatic hepatitis and the worth of preventing it.

The question arises of how these costs should be distributed. If they are spread over the 8 million units of blood transfused, they will increase the price of a unit of blood to approximately $164 and the charges to the average recipient of blood to at least $524, if we assume 3.3 units per patient.

If the beneficiaries of blood services are not limited to those who actually receive blood but include all those who *may* need blood, would it be logical to place all the added cost burden only on the recipients of blood? Clearly it would not. And it would be equally illogical to place the added burden on all hospitalized patients, whether transfused or not. This seems to leave society as a whole, represented by government, as the only source of funds available to absorb the impact of the Kessel proposal.

To state it briefly, the Kessel proposal offers only a promise of achieving, at great additional cost, what is available through an all-volunteer supply at no added cost. Indeed, if one can extrapolate from certain experiences in the voluntary sector, allowing for differences in efficiency of operation, it is conceptually possible that dollar savings could be appreciated by moving to an all-voluntary supply.

The staff of the Council on Wage and Price Stability has made much of the concept of lost opportunity, not only in respect to illness in the victims of post-transfusion hepatitis but also in the diversion of the donor from other activities. The uncertainties in evaluating the time of both paid and voluntary donors make this essentially a fruitless effort. Certainly, it has to be a minor consideration compared with all of the others.

The authors of the National Blood Policy fully recognized that most of the deficiencies in the provision of blood services at the present time stem from failures of organization and from competition where the benefits of competition do not exist. They proposed that the organization involved in blood banking align their relationships in a manner that would ensure resource sharing and more efficient operation. They recognized that there are wide variations in the needs and the opportunities for improvement both within regions and among regions and that ways of meeting these needs would be best designed and implemented by those directly involved.

The authors of the policy also recognized the potential benefits of the donor-recipient link but were aware of the numerous obstacles to full implementation of the principle. At the same time, they saw as a small step the evolution from a mixed volunteer/paid-donor population to an all-volunteer donor population, a step that could be taken *relatively* quickly and at very little, if any, expense and a step that by itself would do more than any other single thing to reduce transfusion-related hepatitis. They intended that the blood-banking community would also fully employ technological advances as they developed, including the best test for the identification of infectious units and donors. They foresaw the possibility that a donor-recipient link might be feasible in certain limited circumstances and considered the desirability of exploring it further, but they could not advocate reliance on it for immediate major gains.

In its attack on the National Blood Policy, the council's staff suggests that an all-voluntary supply is incapable of meeting the demand. This ignores the experience in many parts of the United States and offends those who are now successfully working toward an all-voluntary supply.[9]

If the council's staff truly cannot see how the elimination of any class of blood will be beneficial to consumers, they cannot see that reliance on blood from skid row is dangerous and to be avoided. But there is evidence that they do in fact appreciate the risk, for they suggest the employment of monetary incentives to attract the better socioeconomic groups. At best, their reasoning is confusing.

The opening statement of the National Blood Policy and the first element of the policy itself refer to the need to establish an appropriate ethical climate for the transplantation of human tissues and organs. While there are some members of the blood-banking community who would prefer to ignore this need, there is a substantial body of concerned members who believe very strongly that the need is real and of fundamental importance. This is registered in the statement by the Panel on Blood Resources: "This Panel, recognizing the merits of the lowered cost and increased safety of voluntarily donated blood, is of the opinion that an even more cogent reason for preferring voluntarism is the ethical one. It is important, as noted by Professor Titmuss, to encourage every opportunity for altruism. A society which cherishes the worth of the individual and fosters a high sense of social responsibility cannot set a price on human organs and tissues. Giving blood is regarded as a much needed manifestation of man's humanity to man, to be fostered quite apart from any financial or medical advantages."[10] And yet the council's staff offers the opinion that "blood is a product that is not very different from other consumer goods."

The staff's statement points out that the majority of transfusion-induced hepatitis is attributable to voluntarily donated blood. By failing to acknowledge simultaneously that the commercial sources of blood are disproportionately responsible for transfusion-related hepatitis, it misleads the reader and suggests that the National Blood Policy is attacking the problem inappropriately.

The staff's statement concludes that the label on the blood bag should clearly

[9] Letter to Secretary of Treasury William Simon, from Mr. John Thornton, president of the Richmond Blood Bank, Richmond, Virginia.

[10] Department of Health, Education, and Welfare, National Heart and Lung Institute/ National Institutes of Health, *National Heart, Blood Vessel, Lung and Blood Program; Report of the Blood Resources Panel*, April 6, 1973, pp. 1-5 to 1-7.

and quantitatively indicate the risks of hepatitis from blood. In doing so, it ignores the fact that this cannot be done universally and is impracticable.

In conclusion, one must ask whether the council's staff intended fully to support the concept of blood labeling.

Gordon Tullock

I am an economist and thus am outside the blood-banking or medical professions. As an outsider looking at the American medical system, I see a mess. I begin by observing a cartel of doctors and proceed downhill from there. In fact, almost the only thing one can say in favor of this medical system is that, as far as I can see, other countries have worse systems. On this, Dr. Kellner and I are in general agreement. The medical systems of most other countries do tend to be worse, but there are things that can be done to improve ours.

The blood problem is simply one of many problems in this area. It arises because of third-party payment for the bulk of the expenditures, a set of rather inefficient institutions, and a very powerful (and, by the way, government-organized) cartel.

But turning to the blood market, as far as I can see, the most interesting thing we have been talking about today is the proposal to create a new victimless crime. Consenting adults are not to be permitted to sell blood to each other. I take it we are all in favor of repealing the laws against homosexual acts, prostitution, and so on, but here we have a new victimless crime. It is a little difficult to understand why we should object if two consenting adults engage in this particular act of buying and supplying blood.

There is a peculiar characteristic of what I am told about blood. (I admit frankly that my knowledge of blood has mainly been picked up here and in some casual reading, so I may have misunderstood some of the arguments.) Suppose we have a demand for some commodity or service, in this case blood. Now, we have a supply of voluntary blood, which, we are told, is cheaper than commercial blood. We are also told that the supply is adequate. On the other hand, we observe that some people sell blood at a price which, we are told, is higher than that charged for volunteer blood. Not only that, but we are told that the higher-priced commercial blood is of poorer quality. This is a peculiar set of facts for an economist to observe. One would think that people would not be able to sell blood under these circumstances because cheaper blood of a better quality is obtainable. In addition, one observes that there is a proposal to ban the commercial suppliers. It is as if the presidents of Ford, Chrysler, and General Motors were to say to Congress, we want to have buggies made illegal because they are inferior transportation.

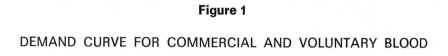

Figure 1

DEMAND CURVE FOR COMMERCIAL AND VOLUNTARY BLOOD

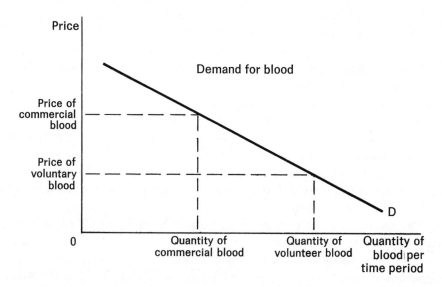

The obvious question to be asked by any economist is why the commercial blood suppliers are not being driven out of business by this superior-quality, lower-cost source. Why is it necessary to seek government intervention? There are several possible explanations that occur to an economist, the obvious one being simply that voluntary blood is *not* sufficient to supply the quantity demanded. Market segmentation would be another. In other words, voluntary blood, today, is producing about 90 to 95 percent of the total demand. Thus, the average purchaser of blood—by this, I do not mean the patient; I mean the hospital or the blood bank—attempts to acquire as much cheap high-quality blood as he can and then supplements it by purchasing the more expensive poorer-quality blood. If this is, in fact, the situation, then, making commercial blood unavailable would create a small, but noticeable, shortage of blood.

There is a possibility that for some reason this would increase the volunteer supplies. I was impressed by Professor Drake's empirical studies, and it does appear that it may be possible to push volunteerism harder. However, it is not clear why that harder push has not already occurred.

Some people representing the blood-banking industry are trying to eliminate their competition. This is not surprising. As it happens, I am a "volunteer" donor in another industry. As you know, since 1932 banks have stopped paying people for depositing money in their checking accounts. Bankers will tell you that the reason for this is, of course, to protect the depositors, and they will give you

153

elaborate rationalizations. They are very sincere about it, and I do not think they are consciously lying. The fact remains that they had Congress pass a law making their principal raw material free. They have not succeeded in totally eliminating competition, but Congress has helped them a good deal. As an economist, I automatically think that when someone asks Congress to eliminate his competitors he must do so from a desire to lead a quiet life. The great advantage for a monopoly is not profit because monopolies are not all that profitable in the long run. However, management finds life easier when competition is gone. This reason would occur to any economist as a possible explanation of why some blood bankers want to eliminate the commercial sector.

It is only a possible explanation. I would need to know much more about the industry than I now do before I would be able to say with certainty that this is true. It is difficult to be sure whether the argument bankers advance for making us voluntary donors of checking accounts is the one that they honestly believe. Their arguments for this law are not totally silly. A number of intelligent students have bought it at one time or another.

The second piece of evidence suggesting that there are efforts to eliminate competition in the blood market comes indirectly from the proposal to establish regional groups and to coordinate blood capacity. I am an outsider, but I do recognize something that is similar to what has happened in other areas of American society. For a number of years, various people have been worried about the existence of the messy pattern of local governments we have in the United States and have sought to coordinate it in order to increase efficiency. The arguments for the establishment of regional governmental units look, superficially, very good, and for a long time I was in favor of most of these measures. In retrospect, we have been able to study this more carefully, and it turns out that when you put a series of these messy organizations together into one large efficient-looking group, output does not improve. On the other hand, taxes increase, the number of employees increases, and the salaries of the senior administrators increase. This has led to the conclusion that the actual motive of the people behind centralization—probably not at a conscious level—was the desire to acquire a monopoly.

As far as I know, no studies of this sort have been made in the nonprofit area, that is, in the area of charitable agencies. We should look into it; it might be a good subject for a doctoral dissertation if any of you has an interested student. Let us see whether an organization—the United Fund or a regional blood center, for example—did not have somewhat that same kind of effect when it was set up. I suspect that it did, but this hypothesis needs testing.

Herbert Polesky

Scientific and technological progress in medicine have been accompanied by a loss in the all-important "art" of medicine. Too frequently, we professionals become enamored of the tools available to us and lose sight of important aspects of the personal relationship between the health-care provider and the patient. Similarly, it appears to me that the health-care planners, government officials, and professors have become so involved with social theory that they have forgotten the importance of individual variables. In meeting patient and community needs one is not dealing with problems that have exact answers.

Professor Drake has pointed out that the current pluralistic system for recruiting blood donors is remarkably successful. The many approaches used have been able to respond to an unpredictable demand complicated by constraints of biologic safety and variables in supply over which the blood bank has little control. The level of service is such that most physicians pay no more attention to the blood supply than to the water supply.

In his paper and presentation Professor Drake has attempted to classify various donor-recruitment systems. He points out that in spite of different ideologies, such as community versus individual responsibility, the recruitment message conveyed to the donor is relatively similar. To the recruiter and often to the donor, individual or family need is most often the motivating force. In my own experience very few people are willing to designate their donation or to be recalled to donate for something as vague as "community service"; yet when a donor is called to meet the needs of a specific patient (more often than not unknown to the donor) the response is excellent and immediate. In spite of or because of the emotional significance of blood implied by religious and cultural beliefs, most people will donate for tangible reasons if it is made convenient for them to donate.

Professor Wallace, after pointing out certain assumptions that tend to ignore historical facts, has shown us fifty-seven measures he would apply to evaluate the performance of a regional blood system. He advocates regionalization as a solution for the problems of a pluralistic system that operates, according to him, on a "best effort basis with minimum expense or expenditure of financial resources."

One assumption that Professor Wallace has failed to state is that he thinks the collection of data and comparison among regions are essential to change. On this point I cannot agree with him. I do agree that responsible management will base decisions on performance criteria and that these should be subjected to peer review locally and perhaps nationally. I favor coordination of services and resource sharing to avoid unnecessary and at times costly duplication. I am opposed to large monopolistic systems of which the initial benefits all too often are soon counterbalanced by deterioration in services and rising costs.

Though performance criteria are useful, it is difficult to use them as absolutes

155

since they will not account for deliberate trade-offs to reach a management objective. For example, it may be more efficient in a narrow sense to use the same donors repeatedly, but a blood program involving a larger donor base which is less efficient may be more desirable in terms of broad social policy.

I have heard little here about the advantages of competition. Yet I have seen two blood programs operating in the same metropolitan area work together to meet patient needs, despite their rival philosophies, and spur each other to provide better services. Dr. Wallace also fails to consider the main problem in any regional system, which I see as arising from personalities and power. What would he do with a large institution whose director justified continuing a competing blood program on the basis of a teaching function and on a cost basis which ignored a large component of indirect tax money?

Regionalization and performance criteria are often advocated because they will control costs. As I look at the proposals to coordinate services I find new bureaucracies, which will impose new costs on programs that are now cost-effective. These seem to have been ignored.

It is always a pleasure to be able to find a few points of agreement with my distinguished colleague, Dr. Kellner. I must agree that blood banking is a dynamic field that has been and is responsive to patient needs. I further agree that the numerous advances made in the past forty years have established a level of service in the United States without equal. All is not perfect, but we have made available the various components needed to support revolutionary changes in patient care.

Dr. Kellner finds that the single most important problem facing us is the ideological question of who is to be responsible for blood policy. On the one hand, he states that it is archaic to keep track of who gives for whom, while on the other hand he sees the need for detailed statistics on the quantity of blood collected and its distribution as an essential cornerstone for the implementation of the National Blood Policy. My own conviction, as I have stated, is that individual and family responsibility are important facets of donor motivation. Blood assurance and the nonreplacement fee provide a useful means of donor recognition and help keep costs down for those who participate without putting an excessive cost or pressure on those who choose not to have their friends or family donate. Through the American Association of Blood Banks Clearinghouse System, which makes it possible to donate in one area for the benefit of someone elsewhere, we have maximized opportunities for replacement. To prevent inequities for the occasional "blood indigent," blood banks such as mine have created special accounts with extra credits to help those without friends and relatives. It amazes me that Dr. Kellner is just now discovering that one can provide replacements for the first three units of blood used by a Medicare patient. That was the whole idea behind the deduction, and in many areas nonreplacement fees are not collected not only for the first three units but also for additional units if the bureaucrats are willing.

Dr. Kellner states that the second problem is voluntarism. I am personally committed, for both fiscal and social reasons, to an all-voluntary donor system. I am concerned that the issues of safety and voluntarism have been confused and that Dr. Meyers and the Bureau of Biologics think that labeling will have an impact on this.

In discussing the problem of obtaining blood and components from an all-voluntary donor population, Dr. Kellner has touched on the issue that I think should have been his number-one priority, that is, the plasmapheresis industry. The policy makers at HEW continue to attack unjustly the segment of the blood-bank complex that is currently meeting the needs of patients and ignore the unsavory practices carried out on the skid rows of most metropolitan areas. I really wonder who is looking out for the public's interest. Trying to meet the needs for plasma products from volunteers will require much effort directed at increasing the utilization of blood components and improving the uses of these plasma derivatives.

I agree with Dr. Kellner that *good* statistics about blood-bank activity will be useful in making policy decisions. In fact, an essential performance criterion should be to maintain, monitor, disseminate, and discuss operational and fiscal data on a local basis. Disclosure on a local level and the practice of including professional and nonprofessional consumers among the policy makers can help to produce programs to effect needed changes. Central collection of large masses of data from many sources is a costly process which will lead to confusion and inappropriate planning.

I agree with Dr. Kellner's comments on governance. It is important that there be opportunity for meaningful input on a policy level by consumers. Boards composed strictly of medical doctors are no worse than those composed of individuals selected because of their social prominence or their potential contributions to a fund drive. There must also be input at policy and operational levels by the transfusion service directors and patients. We need dialogue with the consumer but also a strong but not dominant component of professional leadership.

Since Dr. Kellner concluded with a discussion of regionalization I must again comment on this controversial issue. Local responsibility defined by patient-care patterns would be ideal; however, in my area (as in New York) one institution gets a number of patients, though none of its blood, from outside the United States. There is no way local volunteers could meet all these "imported" needs. A similar imbalance between service and donor availability occurs in many other areas.

Dr. Kellner claims there are 5,000 separate blood-collecting agencies. I am not sure where he gets his figure, but there are probably fewer than 800 separate collecting agencies, and 95 percent of the blood is collected by about 250 banks and their substations. Theoretical models are great for simplifying things to a level bureaucrats can understand; but they do not really take into account the problems of meeting needs in America where geographic facts, patient mobility, population imbalances, and weather affect availability and accessibility.

Louanne Kennedy

I would like to talk a bit about the papers that have been presented as well as my own research, which is specifically concerned with the historical developments in blood banking in the United States.

The papers in Part One appear to blame bureaucratic interference for the defects of the system and, thus, call for the restoration of market competition as the primary influence for adjustment and incremental reform. Specifically, the market adjustment-"reform" proposal assumes that legal rulings provide incentives for efficiency and effectiveness for the blood-collection system.

A contrasting position, that of "administrative rationalization," sees the regulatory divisions of government as providing incentives for the private sector to develop efficient and effective ways of responding to the demands of society. The advocates of this position blame the market competitors for the defects of the system and call for increased administrative regulation and government financing in the control and development of health care. The speakers in this part of today's conference may not represent the second position precisely as I have outlined it, but they are generally responsive, in their studies, to the movement toward administrative reform.

Numerous sociological studies, however, have raised an important problem of increasing reliance upon government regulation; that is, the role of government regulation and funding frequently reinforces, rather than undermines, the private sector.

I would like to speak for a few moments in greater detail about the three papers in Part Three and relate them to my own work. Dr. Drake's paper represents a large investment of both money and time. I would agree with him that the blood-collection system works extremely well in this country; that demand probably determines the amount of blood collected; and that, while there may be shortages, these seem to be small and regional.

He stresses in his paper that the donors he interviewed, in explaining why they donate blood, seem to represent the positions of the providers who do the recruiting and that donors are not troubled by the various ideological positions of the collecting organizations. Although Dr. Drake knows that the attitudes of his donors, in most cases, mesh with the recruiting messages of the collecting facilities, we must await the final results of his research to understand what the effects are on nondonors and ex-donors. It may be that the group of ex-donors and nondonors differs on significant measures of attitude, class, and so on from the donor group. If this is the case then crosspressures, differences between ideology and practice, and/or different messages within the same area are produced by blood-collecting organizations. In areas where several groups espousing differing ideological positions, not necessarily reflected in practice, are collecting blood, a more intense problem potentially exists. It is known that individuals subjected to crosspressures tend not to act. That is, a population exposed to different arguments for giving blood may find it easier not to do anything than to assess the relative merits of various positions.

Dr. Wallace's paper takes a different tack and is concerned with organizational measures of effectiveness and efficiency. Dr. Wallace's work is particularly responsive to the fact that the nonprofit sector has had, in the past, little incentive to develop measures of efficiency and effectiveness. Hospitals especially have been known to not operate responsibly in this regard.

His suggestion to regionalize blood-collection agencies arises from the work of the American Blood Commission. To the extent that it would be possible to use Dr. Wallace's performance measures, it may be possible to lay at rest for the last time discussions of whether or not various systems are more efficient or more effective than others. Previous discussions of performance without supporting data have tended to concentrate only on ideological positions. Thus, opinions have prevailed over facts. I have been working with the Task Force on Donor Recruitment of the American Blood Commission, and I think we can try to use some of the measures that Dr. Wallace has suggested as ways of studying both the social and the economic costs of the various systems of collection.

Dr. Kellner's paper—and, as most of you know, he is a great proponent of the reform movement within blood banking—raises an important point: should blood collection be at the forefront of moves to change the accountability for health care in the United States? He specifically demands an enlarged role for the consumer.

Given the history of government regulation in this country, administrative reform as compared with other modes of change has offered greater opportunity for widespread involvement of consumers in creating rules and guidelines. When we support this model for social change, however, we must remain aware that administrative reform may have negative repercussions. Forceful and concrete precautions must be taken to incorporate *all* interest groups, specifically donor groups and high-volume blood users, as consumer representatives. The important object here is not only that consumer representatives have token memberships on various commissions but also that processes be undertaken that make possible informed citizen participation in decision making. For example, the labeling issue offers an opportunity for consumer involvement. From the time of the first promulgation of the proposal for labeling in the *Federal Register* to its final enactment, consumers and the community at large should be able to reply. This implies an increased role for consumers, who in turn are demanding government responsibility.

My own research on the historical development of blood banking looked specifically into the coordination attempts by the blood-banking community in the 1950s. This attempt at coordination—an agency, known as the Joint Blood Council, which existed between 1955 and 1962—was not able to succeed. An important obstacle to its success was the absence of consumer representation. The Joint Blood Council fought the same battles that are raging today: Who should be responsible for the blood supply, the individual or wider groups within the community? What are the territorial boundaries that define blood-collecting regions for the differing groups? With only provider groups and medical organizations represented within the Joint Blood Council, no change was possible.

The American Blood Commission was founded with pressure from the administrative system, in that one arm of government, the Department of Health, Education, and Welfare, encouraged the private sector to implement a national blood policy. The American Blood Commission was formed by the private sector as the agency to carry out this policy. Unlike the Joint Blood Council, the American Blood Commission contains representation from labor, voluntary associations, and high-volume user organizations, as well as blood providers and professional groups. It therefore offers a unique opportunity to examine a government/private-sector experiment.

In summary, the administrative reform model, through the increased activity of previously unrepresented interest groups and consumers, has increasingly challenged the market "reformers." Representatives of consumers see the administrative model as more responsive to their interests than market reform since it involves at least an administrative apparatus to hear and act upon their demands.

There is a delicate balance between what is and what is needed. This balance precludes dramatic departures from known, safe, and accepted methods. It is an inherent feature of the American political system, with its pluralistic interest group base, that it makes possible only incremental and marginal change. The experiment in government/private-sector interaction that is now being undertaken by the American Blood Commission offers a unique opportunity to examine the range of possibilities that might be achieved through administrative reform.

AUDIENCE PARTICIPATION
AND DISCUSSION

TED MILLER: Dr. Tullock inquired about the necessity of a commercial blood system if enough blood was being provided by the voluntary sector, and Dr. Mitchell suggested a need for federal action. These are nice illustrations of what economists cite as a major disadvantage of charitable organizations, namely, inertia. In papers written ten years ago, for example, the Red Cross said its collection goal, in most regions, was maintenance of its share of the market. It is only recently—and through the mechanism of the National Blood Policy—that the nonprofit blood-banking sector has been goaded to increase its market share. The progress of the Red Cross and of many AABB members has been impressive in that area. Inertia is the probable explanation for the survival of some commercials, and we are moving effectively away from it.

CLARK HAVIGHURST: This question is going to sound facetious and hostile, but it is not meant in that way. Does the attempt to increase the outpouring of volunteer blood really produce the net gain in altruism that its proponents claim? The blood suppliers try to induce guilt in the citizen, who then tries to assuage that guilt by donating blood. In other words, we are willing to accept a zero price and some inconvenience in order to rid ourselves of the guilt feelings that the Red Cross, or whoever, has inspired in us. If this is so, an all-volunteer system may not be morally or ethically superior. It sounds hostile to suggest that the Red Cross is systematically increasing guilt feelings in the society, but, it is a fact that, when the Red Cross asks me to donate blood, I feel guilty if I cannot do it. I also feel somewhat resentful, and that makes me feel even more guilty.

DR. WALLACE: Both of us have had a certain amount of training—you more than I—in economics, and we think about social problems in the way you mentioned. I have observed, however, that some other people do not pattern their behavior and their thinking in that way. I am not always able to understand how they arrive at their conclusions, which are expressed in terms of social values and sociological principles with which I am neither familiar nor sympathetic. These people do not necessarily feel the increased guilt you described. In fact, they may feel a sense of accomplishment.

HERMAN CULL: If what was said by Professor Havighurst is true, then why do we need restrictions on the number of annual donations? Many donors really want to give often, partly because their motivation is altruism.

DR. POLESKY: There is a clear-cut medical reason for restricting donations except for purposes of collecting plasma only. FDA has considered decreasing the legal number of annual donations from the five times that a person can now give to perhaps only three. There are real problems in iron stores and a variety of other things that should be considered. It may be true that the blood supply depends upon multiple donors, but, as Dr. Kellner and I have mentioned, the greater the number of people who become involved in the long run, the better off we will be. We should not encourage multiple donations by a relatively select group of donors. It may be safer in terms of hepatitis transfusion, but in the long run, from the standpoint of public policy, we will benefit from having more people involved.

MR. CORSON: I understand Dr. Havighurst's point to be not only that guilt is the motivation but also that recruiters are instructed to impress upon the donor that he has a responsibility and would be guilty if he failed to meet it.

DR. POLESKY: There is a superb recruitment film produced by the Red Cross and others. It emphasizes the guilt message: Blood is life, pass it on. The theme is subtle, but there is a strong guilt approach to the film's message.

DAN PEARLMAN: It seems to me that this notion of voluntarism has been pursued in an unsophisticated way today. The distinction between being motivated by guilt and being motivated by altruism is a very difficult distinction to make. If the desire is, essentially, to eliminate paying people for their blood, then we need other forms of education and ways of convincing people that certain kinds of things are necessary in the community. If someone suggests that we have a responsibility as a citizen to give blood and we refuse, well, maybe we should feel guilty.

MICHAEL CARDOZO: As a lawyer, I thought I should respond to our other lawyer's question as to whether donors give blood because of guilt. Perhaps that is the reason I have given blood, but I did not think my reasons for giving blood were different from my reasons for giving financial donations to charitable causes. As we know, many charities read off the names of donors in public to make those not named feel a little guilty. If guilt is behind the giving of blood, the same guilt is behind other kinds of charitable donations. It is an obligation, a responsibility of blood bankers, to educate those consumers who are interested in being educated. I am afraid I agree with Dr. Mitchell that such attitudes as Dr. Polesky's are archaic.

162

DR. DRAKE: There are two points I would like to make. One is a comment on the guilt issue, and the other is a brief response to Aaron Kellner, who attributed to me something I never said.

I have considerable experience in studying the attitudes and decision processes of citizens with regard to blood donation. When we think about the guilt issue, as it is sometimes called by the economists, another question occurs to me— Whose model of people should we use, our model or their model? My survey work often asks a subject to tell in his own words the reasons or thoughts associated with his decision to give blood or not to give blood or why he made his first donation, and so on. Even though the subjects usually respond anonymously on self-administered instruments, the guilt notion, by that or any other name, almost never appears.

There is always room for interpretation on such matters. If a person responds that blood donation fulfills a social responsibility, I see no advantage in describing this as guilt. It is true, of course, that the promotional messages of the blood services influence what the person interprets as social responsibility.

My surveys have included another question relative to the guilt issue, namely whether the pressure on the public to donate blood is too little, about right, or too much. If most responses are "too little" or "about right," then guilt seems less of an issue than it might be. The final statistics on this are not in yet, but there is no indication that the general public (including donors) believe they are subject to undue pressure to give blood.

In replying to Aaron Kellner, I never said that ideology is not important. In fact, I have a strong preference for one of the four ideologies I described. I did say that nonideological measures—measures of medical quality and economic performance—will not allow us to resolve the ideological issues. Even if we decided to adopt the system that scored best by the performance measures, it is unlikely that a single ideology would dominate others in terms of performance. Ideological issues have to be settled ideologically. I am convinced of the merits of a particular ideology, but if you happen to have another set of beliefs that are as deeply rooted as mine I have no way whatever to make you see things my way. Therefore, I have to accept your ideology as one that is appropriate for you. But I did not say that ideology is beside the point.

DAVID ENNIS: Dr. Polesky believes there is a form of art in blood banking. I tend to agree with that, but there is also a bit of theatrics. Sometimes I would rather have certain doctors performing in our local theatrical groups than sticking me with a needle.

I would like to address Dr. Kellner's comments, but unfortunately he will not be able to hear them.* He did a fantastic job of including all the characteristics

---

* Editor's Note: Dr. Aaron Kellner had to leave the conference before these comments were made. Because he was unable to reply to Mr. Ennis's comments, portions of Dr. Kellner's subsequent correspondence with Mr. Ennis are included in Appendix A.

that Dale Carnegie recommends for a public address: love, emotions, human appeal. I would like to discuss a few of them.

Love—in New York City? I just wonder how much love there is within the population of New York. If there is such a great deal of love in New York City—so much that the people are willing to roll up their sleeves, altruistically, and give blood—I wonder why that city imports blood from outside of the United States. Concern for the elderly is warranted, and I agree completely with this concern. But age does not denote bankruptcy or indigence. I would imagine that in New York City there are more people under age sixty-five on the welfare rolls than over sixty-five.

Dr. Kellner also mentioned that some individuals live alone, far from their children. Interestingly enough, the AABB created a clearinghouse for just this reason some twenty years ago. In the last fiscal year, more than 300,000 credits were transferred through that network because people in one part of the country wanted to replace blood in another part of the country.

Dr. Kellner said that disclosure was important to him, and disclosure is also important to me, not only disclosure of financial data but also disclosure of data on blood supply and income. On several occasions I have unsuccessfully tried to obtain statistics on Euroblood.* Dr. Kellner recommended that I write the ten largest regional centers for their financial statistics, and I plan to do that, and I also plan to ask him for his information on Euroblood.

The problems with blood banking are numerous and complex, and Dr. Kellner has made some fine points with which I do not disagree. But, as I recall, the article that appeared in *Reader's Digest*—an extremely good article about the New York Blood Center—disclosed no importation of blood from foreign countries.[1] For Dr. Kellner to advocate open disclosure and to disseminate such statements from his public relations department is somewhat inconsistent.

DICK WALKER: Since there are many economists with us today, I want to remind everyone of something that many people overlook—at least that many blood bankers overlook.

I am totally committed to an all-voluntary blood system in this country, and the American Association of Blood Banks is committed to it as well. Although we can accomplish the goal of an all-volunteer blood system, we should not

---

* Editor's Note: Euroblood refers to the red blood cells obtained from donors in a number of Central European countries under a license of the United States Bureau of Biologics. Approximately 1 million units are collected annually in foreign countries for the plasma portion of blood, and, presumably, the red cells would otherwise be discarded. The New York City Blood Center imported approximately 100,000 units of red blood cells in 1975. The New York City Blood Center has the BOB license, and most of the imported Euroblood is used in the New York City area. Some Euroblood is transshipped to other parts of the country.

[1] W. S. Ross, "Better Way to Bank Blood: New York's Blood Center," *Reader's Digest*, vol. 106 (May 1975), pp. 152-56.

deceive ourselves into thinking that this will cost less than the mixed system we now have. Several blood bankers have stated that they have switched from a paid-donor system to an all-voluntary system and discovered that it costs less. These blood bankers fail to consider that the full-time paid recruiter generally designates two to four employees of a company to organize company-wide blood donations. To do this, these employees often spend many hours making telephone calls on company time. The other employees donate their blood on company time, and, depending on where they live, they may receive time off for this purpose. We call this "voluntarism." Many employees who donate on company time would not do so on their own time. Many people equate voluntarism with altruism, but the fact that people are "volunteering" their blood does not mean they are altruistic.

I am sure we will go to an all-voluntary system, and we will prove it can be done, but we should not deceive ourselves on cost. We should take into account the total cost to all persons involved. I am not naive enough to think the employer will absorb all of these costs and not pass them on to the consumer. This is important in figuring what it costs to obtain a so-called voluntary donor.

H. C. ROSER: I had not understood Dr. Polesky to state that he was against the collection of information, but rather that he favored the collection of useful information on a comparable basis, within regions, before considering the usefulness of information collected on a national basis.

In this connection, I have this question for Dr. Mitchell. As Professor Kennedy said, although regulation serves to increase competition, it typically serves also to increase costs. It increases costs by requiring the compilation and dissemination of information, by requiring producing units to establish minimum standards for operations that may not reflect consumer needs, and by deferring operations because of the necessity of getting permission to take action. It also increases prices by limiting competition and restricting supply because it removes incentives for investment.

Such cost increases should be justified by certain compensating social benefits that are achieved. Would it be worthwhile, considering that regulation typically increases costs, to require that, before the FDA or HEW issues new regulations, a regulatory economic impact statement be filed, as is done in the environmental field? Then there would be an opportunity for a full evaluation of the costs and benefits associated with proposed regulatory activity?

DR. MITCHELL: The law already requires the Council on Wage and Price Stability and the Food and Drug Administration to do that.

MARIETTA CARR: I understand that Dr. Solomon stated at another meeting recently that if the regulatory cost was not in the neighborhood of $100 million, it was not considered to have any impact. Is that correct?

165

JOEL SOLOMON: The executive order requires the fixing of an inflationary impact assessment on every regulation that comes out of the agency. We are not required to develop an intensive inflationary impact statement unless the impact will increase the total costs of the product by $100 million or more.

BERNICE HEMPHILL: I think a conference like this has been meaningful for many people. The current blood system in this country has been able to provide services for more than thirty-five years thanks to people willing to be blood donors no matter what recruitment philosophy has been promoted at local levels. I have trouble, therefore, in understanding the relevance of individual responsibility versus community responsibility. If I wish to give my blood for a friend or relative, to predeposit it, or to be paid for it, that is my right of choice as an individual. The blood I give, however, helps the community.

What was said today is that the blood system can function in more than one way. To the people who could not be here today—the professionals in the field— we have said that, whatever the methodology at the "grass roots," the blood system will continue serving the needs of the people as long as it provides safe and adequate blood.

It is my wish that blood banking continue to operate on the basis of what is good at the individual and community levels. I would also like to increase, rather than terminate, relationships such as the interorganizational agreement between the AABB and the American Red Cross, which are in the best interest of the American people.

AFTERWORD

David B. Johnson

One is hesitant to attempt to summarize the proceedings of a conference in which widely divergent views have been expressed and in which time limitations have prevented the thorough discussion of some topics. However, on a few topics there was fairly general agreement. These deserve to be spotlighted.

- Despite the widespread application of the most sensitive third-generation post-transfusion hepatitis tests, there has been only a 50 percent reduction in PTH cases. This has led medical researchers to conclude that there are viruses other than the known types A and B which cause PTH. According to Dr. Gocke, there are no techniques available for the detection of these other viruses.

- Commercial blood, as currently procured in the United States, appears to cause post-transfusion hepatitis at an average rate greater than the average rate for blood procured from so-called voluntary sources. However, for some commercial blood the rate of PTH incidence appears to be lower than the average PTH rate for voluntary blood.

- Blood-collection programs are characterized by numerous practices such as blood insurance, nonreplacement fees, credits, predeposit, and community responsibility by which these programs can be identified as subscribing to one of the two distinct ideologies, community responsibility and individual responsibility. In practice, however, the distinction between these pure ideologies is blurred; blood centers and hospitals often employ techniques and procedures associated with both ideologies. As Alvin Drake pointed out, the availability of blood is generally unrelated to the patient's blood coverage and financial situation and many front-line recruiters for community-responsibility programs employ individual-responsibility messages.

- Apart from the quality of blood, there is little evidence to support the charge that the blood market is serving the American public poorly. All participants agreed that seldom are there general shortages of blood or routine postponements of operations because of a lack of blood. Except in isolated geographical areas and during occasional temporary shortages, the current system seems to be yielding enough blood to supply the increasing demand.

- If strict or fault liability were applied to blood, the quality control of commercial blood and the average quality of transfused blood could be improved. The difficult problem lies in determining the relative economic and social costs of the improved commercial system as compared with the cost of the voluntary system. Ian Mitchell presented some interesting data which were not challenged during the conference and which showed that improved commercial blood would be more expensive.

- Accurate and reliable data on the blood market are improving but they are far from satisfactory. It was anticipated that the various task forces of the American Blood Commission would soon suggest ways to improve data collection and availability.

- Although the National Blood Policy commits the nation to an all-volunteer blood system, there was considerable disagreement about the definition of a volunteer.

Numerous other points of significant interest and impact were made by the participants, but they were more controversial than those listed above. One important aspect of this conference was the number of issues it raised and the outline it provided for further thought and research. Taking a modicum of editorial liberty, I would like to discuss some areas for research that were mentioned during the conference or occurred to me as I listened to our proceedings and which, in my personal view, are significant. My raising of these issues does not imply that I support a particular position.

Commercialism: Procurement versus Distribution

One important distinction not emphasized by the conference participants is that commercialism in blood procurement does not necessarily imply commercialism in blood distribution. Doctors treating indigent medical patients, for example, do not volunteer their services. They are paid for their services through the Medicaid or Medicare programs rather than by the patient. Similarly, the fact that payments are made to blood providers does not necessarily mean that low-income individuals or others will have to pay for the blood they receive. As some participants pointed out, there are advantages in requiring recipients to pay for blood just as they pay for other goods. However, *if* ethical or other considerations preclude the pricing of blood to patients, the payments could be made by local or federal governments or by some charitable agency. It is important to recognize that the concern expressed by several speakers about the inability of poor or elderly patients to pay for blood refers not to the procurement of blood but to the pricing policies applied to its allocation or distribution. In a commercial blood system, the two sides can be easily separated.

It is interesting to note that the procurement and distribution sides of the blood market *cannot* be easily separated from that part of the blood market which is characterized by the replacement fee. Although many health insurance plans cover the replacement fee and many hospitals do not require the old or the poor to pay the replacement fee, the two sides of the market cannot be analytically separated because the central thesis of the replacement-fee philosophy is that blood can be procured primarily by placing the responsibility on those who have received (or may receive) blood. It is ironic that some who express concern about the burden placed upon patients prefer to move toward a voluntary system, with replacement or responsibility fees, and away from a commercial system that could eliminate this burden if social policy so required.

Definition of a Volunteer

A second issue, which will have a wide impact not only in the blood market but also in the health industry and in the entire third market (the private but not-for-profit sector), is the definition of a volunteer and, subsequently, the identification and determination of the opportunity costs of volunteering. Some blood bankers would define a volunteer as one who received no monetary compensation for his blood. Thus, a donor who participated in a blood insurance or assurance plan or who donated blood to avoid a replacement fee, to obtain time off from work, to participate in a raffle, or to obtain tickets to a sporting event would be classified as a volunteer. Few economists would accept this definition of a volunteer because they recognize that the quid offered in exchange for the quo need not be a monetary payment but can be a payment "in kind." Many employees, including executives, doctors, and university presidents, receive income in other than monetary payments. Stock options, large offices, homes, use of the company (university) car, insurance policies, and paid vacations are forms of payments. We do not classify an executive who receives all or part of his compensation through such means as a complete or partial volunteer. Similarly, to classify a blood donor who receives payment "in kind" as a volunteer is not only to misuse the King's English but also to cause misleading impressions and faulty reasoning.

Perhaps some of the terminological confusion can be traced to the desire of the Department of Health, Education, and Welfare and the Bureau of Biologics, among others, to differentiate between high- and low-risk blood. This distinction was made on the basis of volunteer versus commercial donor. If one recognizes that some commercial blood (qua monetary payment) is high-quality blood, the distinction between commercial and volunteer (broadly defined) can be defended on strictly medical grounds. By making exceptions for the obviously high-quality commercial blood and by eliminating the remaining commercial blood for which monetary payments are made under the current system, a voluntary blood system can obviously produce, overall, higher-quality blood. The explanation is simply that under current practices the skid row types—drug addicts, prostitutes, and so on—would be largely eliminated. But if one is to attempt to differentiate between high- and low-quality blood, it would be just as easy to label all blood higher quality or lower quality or to label the social and economic characteristics of the donor and to dispense with the volunteer-commercial distinction.

The broad definition of the volunteer donor is even less useful when one considers the social and ethical aspects of blood policy. If altruism is to be the motivating force in the procurement of blood, then donors receiving extra time off, even time off from work while donating, or insurance against their future blood needs in exchange for their donations should not be called volunteers. When used in this social and ethical sense, the volunteer-commercial distinction becomes a red herring. Perhaps the debate should focus on altruism versus incentivism, with an altruist defined as one who donates on his own time with no selective incentive such as additional time off from work, blood assurance or replacement, or any gifts or payments. An incentive-motivated individual, obviously, is one who receives some payment in money or in kind, including blood insurance, gifts, or additional vacation days.

Even an apparently altruistic blood-procurement system *might* be ethically undesirable because, as Clark Havighurst pointed out, individuals may be coerced into donating blood. A brief discussion of the major integrative mechanisms may place the role of social pressure in analytical focus.

There are at least three integrative mechanisms in society. The first and most thoroughly developed at the theoretical level is the private market, in which individuals sell or exchange goods for other goods or for the common denominator of money. The second is the political market, in which individuals direct the allocation of resources through the ballot box. The third is the charity market, in which individuals make allocative and production decisions neither through the ballot box nor through the price mechanism. What motivates individuals within the private market is the price mechanism;[1] the motivating factor in the political market is the threat of fines or imprisonment if taxes are not forthcoming. The motivating variable in the charity market is unclear. It is certainly possible that some individuals are genuine altruists; it is also possible that social pressure will induce them to "donate."

If a significant portion of blood is procured through a system which utilizes group or personal competition or social pressure, then such a system is ethically less desirable to many, including this author, than one in which incentives, including monetary payments, are extensively utilized. This problem of social pressure

---

[1] The existence of a positive price for a commodity such as blood does not remove the possibility that donors are altruists. An individual may value the time, effort, and discomfort at fifty dollars but charge only twenty dollars for the unit of blood he donates. The remaining thirty dollars per unit corresponds to the altruistic component of his donation.

is not peculiar to the blood market; it exists in all aspects of the so-called charity market.

The social-pressure thesis is not amenable to simple empirical testing. Individuals are unlikely to perceive the effects of social pressure operating even in their personal cases. If they do perceive the application of social pressure they have no incentive to reveal it to an investigator but they do have a positive incentive to conceal it if doing so makes them appear "socially conscious." Thus, it is not especially surprising that Professor Drake did not find the existence of social pressure in his empirical studies.

One possible way to test the social-pressure hypothesis is to examine thoroughly the actual recruiting techniques employed by the blood centers. If donors are obtained openly from the entire community and not from certain church, labor, or other organizations in which social pressure and individual or group competition can be employed and if they receive no individual incentives such as assurances of future blood provision, public recognition, money, or gifts for their donation, then one might conclude that such donors are primarily motivated by altruism. On the other hand, if the "volunteer" donors are obtained through work groups or church, fraternal, or community organizations, past research has suggested that social pressure is likely to be more prevalent.[2]

Even if one could determine that 100 percent of blood donors are true altruists, one could not immediately accept the conclusion that altruism is an efficient basis for a procurement system. As Professor Tullock mentioned in his paper, love is a scarce resource which must be allocated efficiently. If an individual contributes blood in place of volunteering some other public service, the opportunity cost of his donation might be higher than the cost of procuring a unit of equal-quality blood through direct monetary or in-kind incentives. For example, a housewife might donate a pint of blood that could have been obtained on the commercial market for $25. If she had not donated the blood she might have spent five hours as a volunteer nurse with her services valued at $100. Thus, the volunteer sector is obtaining services valued at $25 by forgoing services valued at $100. A major deficiency in the third market is that there exists no mechanism for determining the relative values of different altruistic acts or for generating suitable incentives or information to direct scarce altruism into the areas where it is needed most.

In his paper on performance measures, Professor Wallace suggested criteria to be used in the evaluation of blood-center efficiency. But even if we had efficiency, narrowly interpreted, at the individual-operating-unit level, there would

---

[2] Social pressure is more effective in small groups than in large ones, and many charitable funds attempt to segment a large community into smaller groups for fund-raising purposes. See David B. Johnson, *Some Fundamental Economics of the Charity Market*, Ph.D. dissertation, University of Virginia (1968) and T. R. Ireland and D. B. Johnson, *The Economics of Charity* (Blacksburg, Virginia: Public Choice Society, 1970).

still be a need for a mechanism to integrate efficiency among all blood centers and other charitable agencies and a useful definition of *volunteer*.

The above discussion should not be interpreted as a criticism of an all-volunteer blood-procurement system. As a nation we would be fortunate indeed if individuals freely supplied the blood needed by their fellow citizens. But we should not rush into a system which defines *volunteer* in a misleading and analytically incorrect way, which imposes higher costs than some other system, or in which the most scarce of all resources—love of one's fellow man—is inefficiently allocated.

A Uniform System of Accounts

Economic, medical, legal, and social analysis can be very useful approaches to the blood market but, as in many other industries, the final answers will depend upon empirical data. Some of these data, such as the opportunity costs of volunteer donors, have to be based on information largely external to a blood center. Other information, however, will have to be obtained from the internal records of blood centers and hospitals.

Important empirical questions for which internal data are required include the following: What are the costs of operating bloodmobiles, satellite-, and central-collection centers? What components are used in costing the blood supplied the hospitals? Do these components, such as research and cross-matching, vary among blood centers? What is the processing fee and how is it calculated? Why is the total price charged by some commercial blood banks less than the processing fee charged by volunteer blood centers? Do different blood types sell at varying prices? Are they cost-related? Is peak-period pricing utilized, or should it be utilized? Are "profits" earned and then used to subsidize other areas of an agency's activities? How are fixed costs allocated to units of blood?

These are just a sample of the questions which empirical investigators would like to ask. However, the current accounting systems of blood centers and hospitals would make the answers to such questions unavailable or meaningless because blood centers do not use a uniform accounting system.[3] Hence, it would appear that many social-policy decisions will have to await the introduction of a uniform system of accounts for the most fundamental aspects of blood banking. Perhaps this suggestion could be pursued by the American Blood Commission.

Euroblood

Dave Ennis raised a point during the afternoon session concerning the Euroblood market which was subsequently answered by Aaron Kellner in the correspondence

---

[3] The Red Cross has recently introduced a uniform accounting system for its fifty-eight blood centers.

reprinted in Appendix A. If the citizens of Europe are willing to provide blood to the citizens of the United States more cheaply than it can be procured here, then blood should be imported. Dr. Kellner reports that in 1975 more than 20 percent of the New York center's blood collections were Euroblood. Before its importation into the United States, this blood, collected in Europe under a Bureau of Biologics license, was used only for plasma, the red cells being discarded. Now, under the Euroblood program, the red cells are sent to the United States.

This importation of blood appears to work well for the New York Blood Center by improving the average quality of blood and by lowering the average cost. It would seem advantageous to extend the Euroblood program to large blood centers in other parts of the country.

The mutual advantages of international trade are not limited to the Euroblood market; they are also applicable to blood or plasma procured from Latin America or Africa. There has been, perhaps, an unwarranted criticism of American drug companies' obtaining plasma from Latin Americans. Although the price paid for plasmapheresis in Latin America may appear to be low by our standards, the citizens of Latin America obviously believe they benefit or they would not participate. If repeated donations pose a threat to the health of the donors, then arrangements should be made with the host country to require the companies to inform them of these potential risks. The answer is not to prohibit international trade in blood or plasma.

The Plasma Submarket

The administrative, legal, and medical distinctions between the two submarkets of the blood market—whole blood and plasma—have not been sharply delineated. This conference was directed primarily at the whole-blood market, and virtually all participants discussed solely that segment. However, whether one agrees with Dr. Kellner's suggestion that the plasma submarket should be reorganized along noncommercial lines or not, this issue looms on the horizon. Whether as a result of future regulation by government or as a result of decisions by nonprofit entities, any reorganization of the plasma/drug-derivative segment of the blood market will have broader ramifications than those which have occurred in or have been proposed for the whole-blood market.

Appendix A

APPENDIX A
Aaron Kellner's Response to David Ennis and Summary of Ennis's Response to Kellner

June 24, 1976

Dear Mr. Ennis,

I regret very much that circumstances compelled me to leave the meeting on "Blood Policy: Issues and Alternatives" before you made your comments, which I have read in the verbatim transcript. I would have relished the opportunity to reply to you directly and before a live audience. There are few things I enjoy more than disseminating publicly the facts about Euroblood. Let me now reply seriatim to the points you raised at the meeting.

1. *"Love" in New York.* The figures in the accompanying table demonstrate that New Yorkers contribute vast amounts of blood; indeed, they contribute more blood voluntarily than do the residents of any other metropolitan area in the world.

2. *The elderly and the clearinghouse.* New York, like every other large city, has thousands of old people who are alone and who live at or below the poverty level. As a group they need and use large amounts of blood, proportionately more than any other segment of the population. Those who have family and friends should of course be requested (not coerced) to donate blood. However, to pervert an instrumentality of government designed to help the elderly into a cruel economic bludgeon would demonstrate an unconscionable lack of humanity.

The clearinghouse and the 300,000 transferred credits that you cited, when carefully analyzed, turn out to be irrelevant. Only a small percentage of the 300,000 credits were for the elderly, and only a small percentage of that small percentage represents newly donated blood. The bulk of the 300,000 credits were essentially useless pieces of paper representing blood debits and credits that added little or nothing to the blood supply. The raison d'être of the clearinghouse is the

---

Editor's Note: During an audience participation period, Dr. Aaron Kellner, director of the New York Blood Center, departed before David Ennis, assistant executive director of the Delaware Blood Bank, raised several questions pertaining to the New York Blood Center, Euroblood, and the concept of community responsibility. When Dr. Kellner received the transcript of the meeting, he wrote to Mr. Ennis.

Most of Dr. Kellner's letter is published here because, had he been present when Mr. Ennis made his comments, he would have had the opportunity to reply. In addition, Dr. Kellner presents information about the Euroblood market that both critics and advocates should find interesting. Mr. Ennis's reply to Dr. Kellner is also briefly summarized.

nonreplacement fee, and for Medicare patients that punitive fee only compounds the rip-off. I must remind you, too, that the figure of 300,000 you cite is less than one-third of the amount of blood that is outdated and thrown away in this country each year. There is a means of demonstrating our concern for the elderly, and it is not the clearinghouse.

3. *Euroblood*. The transcript quotes you as saying that you have tried on several occasions to obtain statistics about Euroblood and were unsuccessful. Truly an amazing statement. I cannot imagine to whom your inquiries were directed. I should think you would go directly to the source. Euroblood has been reported in the news media both here and abroad, and I have openly revealed all the operating details and statistics at national and international meetings. There is nothing secret about it. The following table is a summary of blood collections made between 1972 and 1975 by the Greater New York Blood Program including Euroblood:

AMOUNTS OF BLOOD COLLECTED FOR GREATER NEW YORK BLOOD PROGRAM, BY ORIGIN, 1972-1975

| Year | Blood Collected (in units)[a] | | | Percent Euroblood |
	Domestic	Euroblood	Total	
1972	293,879	0	293,879	0
1973	330,976	22,070	353,046	6.25
1974	377,119	70,018	447,137	15.66
1975	417,253	110,658	527,911	20.96

[a] A unit is generally 450 cc or approximately a pint.
Source: New York Blood Center.

I would like to present the following facts about Euroblood:

(a) The blood we refer to by the code name Euroblood would have been collected in any case, the plasma removed, and the red cells discarded. At least 1 million units of voluntarily donated blood are collected each year in central Europe for plasma and the red cells wasted.

(b) Euroblood is collected under our license, approved and inspected by the Bureau of Biologics, using our bags, our donor cards, and our donor-selection and collection standards. All the testing and labeling is done in our laboratories in New York.

(c) Our domestic collections in the New York region have continued to increase progressively and have not been adversely affected by the Euroblood supplementation.

(d) Euroblood is cost-effective, even including air transport, and it helps to lower our average unit cost in New York.

(e) Euroblood is "better" blood; the prevalence of hepatitis B carriers in Euroblood is about half that of blood voluntarily donated in metropolitan areas of the United States. The figures for 1975 are as follows:

PREVALENCE OF HEPATITIS B$_s$AG POSITIVE IN BLOOD USED BY THE GREATER NEW YORK BLOOD PROGRAM, BY ORIGIN, 1975

Origin of Blood	Prevalence per 1000 Units
New York–New Jersey	2.3
Euroblood	1.03
Berne	1.27
Springe	0.44
Rottenburg	0.35
Bad Kreuznach	0.30
Baden Baden	0.35

Source: New York Blood Center.

The rates for 1975 are slightly higher than those for previous years because second-generation testing methods were used for part of 1974 and only third-generation tests in 1975.

4. *The Reader's Digest.* When Walter Ross came to the Blood Center in 1974 for background for his article in the *Reader's Digest*, he was given carte blanche; he was free to delve into any aspect of our operations and to write about anything that interested him and his readers. Nothing was held back. He wrote the story in his own way and in his own words. The omission of Euroblood was his decision, not ours; perhaps he is planning a separate article on that fascinating and productive program. Incidentally, we have large and active programs in genetics, epidemiology, virology, operation research, and transplantation that were not even mentioned in the article. Should I have lodged a complaint with the editor? I should also tell you that for the hundreds of stories and interviews that have appeared about the New York Blood Center, not once have we insisted on the right of prior review.

Sincerely yours,

Aaron Kellner, M.D.
Director
New York Blood Center

Summary of Dr. Ennis's Reply: Dr. Ennis made many of the replacement-fee arguments that were mentioned during the conference; consequently they will not be repeated here. Other arguments he made included the following:

- A system based on individual responsibility does not preclude altruism. Mr. Ennis cited an example of a Delaware couple who required enormous quantities of blood following the delivery of their child in a New York hospital. Through the clearinghouse system, Delaware donors contributed ninety-three pints of blood to this couple.

- The National Blood Policy requires that a *variety* of approaches be utilized in obtaining blood. A purely altruistic blood program may not be sufficient. Mr. Ennis cites the example of Hawaii's Blood Bank, which dropped its replacement fee, only to reinstate it two years later.

- If Euroblood is so good for New York City, why not extend the importation of blood to other parts of the country?

Appendix B

Reprinted for private circulation from THE JOURNAL OF LAW AND ECONOMICS, Volume XVII (2), October, 1974, Copyright 1974, The University of Chicago.

TRANSFUSED BLOOD, SERUM HEPATITIS, AND THE COASE THEOREM*

REUBEN A. KESSEL
University of Chicago

THE late Professor Richard M. Titmuss, in a volume entitled *The Gift Relationship,* delivered a scathing indictment of the system of collecting and delivering blood in the United States by comparing unfavorably the American blood delivery system with the one that prevails in England.[1] The key to Titmuss's objection to our blood delivery system, which utilizes both voluntary and paid donors, is the fact that patients contract hepatitis, more specifically serum hepatitis, substantially more frequently in the United States than in England as a result of blood transfusions.[2] According to Titmuss, about three and one-half per cent of all transfused patients in the United States subsequently contract hepatitis; in England, the corresponding number is under one per cent.[3] This is equivalent to saying that the frequency of hepatitis as a result of transfusion in the United States exceeds England by a factor of about four.

Commercialism in blood procurement—the utilization of paid as an alternative to unpaid (which is not equivalent to Titmuss's altruistic) donors— is held responsible for the higher frequency of transfusion hepatitis in the United States. (It is widely believed that the frequency of hepatitis among recipients of blood from paid donors is roughly ten times greater than it is for unpaid donors.)[4] Commercial donors, according to Titmuss, discourage

---

* The author wishes to acknowledge the assistance of Professor Ronald Coase. An earlier version of this paper was presented at the Industrial Organization Workshop at the University of Chicago.

[1] Richard M. Titmuss, The Gift Relationship: From Human Blood to Social Policy (1971).

[2] There are two types of hepatitis, serum or transfusion (type B) and infectious (type A). These names were derived from beliefs about how these maladies were transmitted which subsequent findings do not wholly support. Hence they have been renamed in a manner that is not suggestive of how they are transmitted or acquired. Both attack the liver. Type B has a substantially longer incubation period, and is more lethal.

[3] Richard M. Titmuss, *supra* note 1, at 146 & 154.

[4] See National Heart and Lung Institute (NHLI) Blood Resources Studies Summary Report 63 (U.S. Dep't Health, Ed. & Welfare, NIH 73-416, June 30, 1972) [hereinafter cited as NHLI Summary Report]. The full NHLI report is published in 3 volumes. Vol. 1: Supply and Use of the Nation's Blood Resource; vol. 2: Regulation of the Nation's

or eliminate voluntary donors; bad blood suppliers drive good blood suppliers out of business. Moreover, he regards malpractice suits as undesirable commercialism which he contends, along with organized medicine in the United States, leads to wasteful "defensive" medicine.[5]

Titmuss also uses economic criteria to compare the "economic efficiency" of the English and American blood delivery systems and finds the American system less efficient.[6] Consequently, Titmuss is less than enamoured with the price mechanism as a means of organizing the production and marketing of blood. Indeed, Titmuss has great reservations about the virtues of the price mechanism for organizing the production and allocation of scarce resources generally; it is his view that the world needs more love and less pecuniary calculation.

The thesis that the price mechanism should not be used for the organization and production of anything arouses the ire of Arrow and Solow.[7] However, they either do not object to or endorse the view that the commercial donor should be outlawed and replaced by the volunteer donor in order to reduce the incidence of hepatitis.[8]

Blood Resource; vol. 3: A Pilot Study of Hemophilia Treatment in the United States (U.S. Dep't Health, Ed. & Welfare, 1973).

[5] Richard M. Titmuss, *supra* note 1, ch. 9, and 197. Although not explicit, it appears that he would attribute "unnecessary" surgery to commercialism in the medical care market. It is unclear whether Titmuss would hold corresponding views about the effects of malpractice suits for lawyers and consulting economists.

[6] A relevant test of Titmuss's hypothesis—that commercialism increases economic inefficiency—is to look for a relationship between the degree of commercialism in an area or region and the measure Titmuss uses to gauge economic efficiency. Titmuss asserts that Seattle has a relatively non-commercial source of blood; hence, if Titmuss is right, an investigation ought to show it to be an area in which blood is efficiently allocated.

[7] See Kenneth J. Arrow, Gifts and Exchanges, in 1 Philosophy & Public Affairs 343 (1972); Robert M. Solow, Blood and Thunder, 80 Yale L.J. 1696 (1971).

[8] Michael H. Cooper & Anthony J. Cuyler, The Price of Blood (Inst. of Econ. Affairs, 1968) advocate thoroughgoing commercialism in the organization and distribution of blood. However, they do not deal with the issue of transfusion hepatitis except for one discussion question following the conclusion of their paper, and a reference to a paper by J. Garrott Allen (& Wynn A. Sayman, Serum Hepatitis from Transfusions of Blood, 180 J. Am. Med. Ass'n 1079 (1962)) who has done as much as anyone to alert the medical profession to the incidence and risks of serum hepatitis.

Another possible exception is Marc A. Franklin who has written two important papers dealing with this subject. They are entitled: Tort Liability for Hepatitis; An Analysis and a Proposal, 24 Stan. L. Rev. 439 (1972); and Hepatitis, Blood Transfusions and Public Action, 21 Catholic Univ. L. Rev. 683 (1972). In the second article, Franklin is mostly concerned with alternative legal and social arrangements for providing blood.

E. R. Jennings, Not All Paid Donors Pose Hepatitis Risks, 2 Lab. Medicine July, 1971, at 8, argues that it is the socio-economic status of donors, not whether or not they are paid, that matters. Hence, the selection of donors, paid or unpaid, ought to be by socio-economic class. He unambiguously disagrees with Titmuss on this critical point.

The NHLI study, vol. 1, *supra* note 4, app. C, at 4 concludes: "The incidence of post-transfusion hepatitis is apparently associated with the specific socio-economic conditions

Arrow points to the absence of a mechanism to equilibrate the quantity of blood demanded with the quantity supplied in Titmuss's explanation of the working of the English system.[9] This is of some relevance because it deals with the principal piece of empirical evidence in Cooper and Cuyler—a survey of blood availability when surgeons wish to operate—which Titmuss dismisses out of hand. Over one-third of the surgeons surveyed reported that they sometimes postpone operations for want of blood.[10]

Support for Cooper and Cuyler's explanation of the equilibrating mechanism appears in a review article by Surgenor:

In England, an order by a physician for a blood transfusion is usually conditional upon the availability of blood. In the United States, this is not so; an order for blood is generally not negotiable by a hospital and must be carried out.[11]

Surgenor does not take seriously Titmuss's conclusion that the English system of blood distribution is more efficient because of the absence of data bearing on the question and the failure by Titmuss to take account of the foregoing ". . . fundamental difference between British and American medical practice."[12]

It is the thesis of this paper that Titmuss can be interpreted in a way which makes his conclusion correct. More specifically, Titmuss can be interpreted as arguing that the mechanism for supplying blood to patients is not responsive to their desires—that too low a quality has been supplied. This has been attributed by Titmuss to excessive commercialism; it is explained here as a consequence of insufficient commercialism. Titmuss is correct for the wrong reason.

The first section of this paper deals with the value of hepatitis-free blood; the second with how a system of blood supply, which is responsive to consumer desires, would operate; the third with why the current system, which is moving towards a wholly voluntary system of blood procurement, has come into existence.

A. THE VALUE OF HEPATITIS-FREE BLOOD

Given the current state of medical technology, there exists no practical way to test effectively for the presence of hepatitis in the blood of all donors.

---

of the donor population rather than with the incentives used in collecting the material." This position is somewhat at variance with what is said on this subject elsewhere in this volume, for example, p. 13, as well as in the summary volume.

[9] Kenneth J. Arrow, *supra* note 7, at 356.

[10] Michael H. Cooper & Anthony J. Cuyler, *supra* note 8, at 17.

[11] D. MacN. Surgenor, Human Blood and the Renewal of Altruism: Titmuss in Retrospect, in 2 Int'l J. Health Sciences, 443, 444 (1972).

[12] *Id.*

The capability of transmitting transfusion hepatitis via blood is detected by testing for the presence of a hepatitis-associated antigen, HBA_g. The best testing method in current use reveals about twenty-five per cent of all hepatitis carriers. Other tests in the wings offer the promise of detecting a maximum of fifty per cent.[13] (There seems to be discreet silence on the question of how much good blood it falsely rejects.) The risk associated with hepatitis rises monotonically with age. It is believed that many infants, particularly infants raised in crowded and relatively unsanitary conditions, incur hepatitis subclinically, that is, no one knows it. By contrast, one study shows that about twenty per cent of those who contract transfusion hepatitis after the age of forty die as a result.[14]

Of the set of transfused patients who manifest symptoms of hepatitis, one HEW report estimates that half convalesce at home for a month without hospital treatment. The other half are hospitalized for about a month and convalesce at home for another month provided they are not among the ten per cent of those hospitalized who die as a result of hepatitis.[15] The costs of (1) subclinical cases, which is estimated to exceed the clinical cases by a factor of five, (2) the transmission of other ailments such as malaria, (3) physician fees, (4) those who never fully recover, estimated to be about equal in number to those who die, and undergo a lifetime of both treatment and sub-par health, and (5) home care are all ignored.[16] For those who never fully recover, their life length is shortened and characterized by tiredness, irritability, lassitude, etc. Clearly hepatitis, unlike warts and athlete's foot or feet, is an extremely costly ailment. Moreover, those who incur this disease typically become more irritable and difficult to live with, a consideration which is not trivial for the marital partners and others associating with hepatitis patients.

The value to patients of high quality blood can be illustrated by very primitive cost calculations. Costs associated with transfusion hepatitis are: (1) for those hospitalized, thirty days at $125 per day taking account of physician fees, laboratory work, etc., which comes to $3,750; (2) the opportunity costs of being out of the labor market, which HEW estimates at $450 a month after adjusting for average participation in the labor market;[17]

[13] See Martin Goldfield, *et al.*, Hepatitis Associated with the Transfusion of HBA_g-Negative Blood, in Hepatitis and Blood Transfusion, Proceedings of a Symposium held at Univ. of Calif. 320 (Girish N. Vyas, Herbert A. Perkins, & Rudi Schmid eds. 1972) [hereinafter cited as Hepatitis and Blood Transfusion].

[14] J. Garrott Allen & Wynn A. Sayman, *supra* note 8, at 1079, 1084.

[15] Posttransfusion Hepatitis: Cases, Deaths, and Costs, in U.S. Dep't Health, Ed. & Welfare, Conference on the National Blood Policy 4 (unpublished reports, 1973).

[16] *Id.* at 1-10.

[17] *Id.* at 5.

(3) home nursing care at $450 per month; (4) treatment for the non-hospitalized at $500; (5) $200,000 as the value of human life which is also used as the cost of being permanently disabled and is obtained from estimates of the value workers place on their lives as inferred from their own behavior.[18] The foregoing implies that the expected costs of hepatitis are $23,225.[19]

The probability of getting hepatitis in the United States as a result of a transfusion of blood seems to depend upon the socio-economic class of the donors, the number of pints involved in a transfusion, and whether or not one has had hepatitis or has natural immunity. The average size of transfusions appears to be rising as a result of the development of open-heart surgery which is a very blood-intensive procedure using up to twenty pints. For open-heart surgery patients transfused with paid donor blood, one study reports about half incurred hepatitis.[20]

An extensive and recently reported study of the incidence of hepatitis among open-heart surgery patients at fourteen so-called university hospital centers contains a body of data useful for estimating the value of a marginal shift in blood sources.[21] These data, reproduced in Table 1, imply that the frequency of symptomatic hepatitis is 8.8 cases per one thousand units of the lowest quality of blood transfused against 2.0 per thousand for the best quality. Hence, a shift from the worst to the best blood implies a reduction in the risk of hepatitis of 6.8 parts per thousand. What would such

[18] Richard Thaler & Sherwin Rosen, Estimating the Value of Saving a Life: Evidence from the Labor Market 36 (Nat'l Bur. Econ. Res., Conf. on Res. in Income & Wealth, Dec. 1, 1973) estimate the value of a human life at $200,000 in 1967 dollars.

[19] The expected costs of hospitalization and inpatient treatment are $1875; death and permanent disability, $20,000; home nursing, $425; absence from the labor market, $675; outpatient medical treatment, $250. These numbers are derived from Richard Thaler & Sherwin Rosen, *supra* note 18; and Posttransfusion Hepatitis, *supra* note 15, except for permanent disability and outpatient medical treatment which are added by the author.

[20] John H. Walsh, *et al.*, Post Transfusion Hepatitis After Open-Heart Operations, 211 J. Am. Med. Ass'n 261 (1970).

[21] George F. Grady, Ann J. E. Bennett, *et al.*, Risk of Posttransfusion Hepatitis in the United States, 220 J. Am. Med. Ass'n 692, tab. 4, at 695 (1972). The reported lethality—eight deaths out of 135 severe cases of hepatitis or 6%—may be at variance with the findings of J. Garrott Allen & Wynn A. Sayman, *supra* note 8. No information is provided on the age of patients other than the fact that those who died were all over sixty. Similarly no information was provided on the average length of hospital stay.

This study surprisingly reported the use of pooled plasma and fibrinogen. Since one contaminated unit in a pool is sufficient to contaminate the entire pool, it is difficult to reconcile this practice with concern for the welfare of patients. (The incidence of hepatitis requiring hospitalization of a week or more was 6% for those receiving plasma and 16% for the recipients of fibrinogen.) Multiple-donor plasma was removed from inter-state commerce by government order in 1968; however, multiple donor fibrinogen continues to be used to the puzzlement of the authors of this paper. Titmuss viewed with horror the existence of such pooling and argued that it is absent in England. See Richard M Titmuss, *supra* note 1, at 149.

a reduction be worth? If the expected costs of hepatitis are $23,000, a reduction in the probability of getting hepatitis by one part in one thousand is worth $23, and a shift from the lowest to the highest quality source would be worth approximately 156 additional dollars per unit, that is, 156 additional dollars above and beyond what is now the cost of the lowest quality blood. The foregoing calculation is highly sensitive to the assumptions made about the opportunity costs of time, cost of home nursing care, the magnitude of the blood quality differences that exist, and above all the value of a marginal extension of life.

The evidence presented by Titmuss to support his contention that the frequency of transfusion hepatitis is greater in the United States leaves something to be desired. Differences in standards of reporting, size of transfusions, use of blood derivative products, representativeness of the sample observed, and the definition of commercialism are all problems largely ignored.

TABLE 1

POSTTRANSFUSION VIRAL HEPATITIS ACCORDING TO SOURCE OF DONOR BLOOD

	Average No. of Units of Blood[a] Per Patient	Patients at Risk	Hepatitis Cases		
			All	Symptomatic	Severe
In Patients Receiving All Transfusions From a Single Category					
Group 1: Red Cross donors only	7.4	715	10(1.4%)	10(1.4%)	9(1.3%)
Group 2: Other volunteer donors only	6.4	354	6(1.7%)	6(1.7%)	6(1.7%)
Group 3: Paid donors, known to transfusionist	6.3	396	13(3.3%)	12(3.0%)	11(2.8%)
Group 4: Prebottled blood from paid donors	4.9	625	33(5.3%)	27(4.3%)	19(3.0%)
In Patients Receiving Transfusions From Mixed Sources					
Groups 1, 2, 3 above but no prebottled blood from paid donors	9.3	1,550	35(2.3%)	35(2.3%)	28(1.8%)
Prebottled blood from paid donors and some blood from groups 1, 2, or 3	8.1	1,314	57(4.3%)	47(3.6%)	38(2.9%)
Single Sources and Mixed Sources					
Totals	7.7	4,954[b]	154(3.1%)	137(2.8%)	111(2.2%)

Source: George F. Grady, Ann J. E. Bennett, *et al.,* Risk of Posttransfusion Hepatitis in the United States, 220 J. Am. Med. Ass'n 692 (1972).

[a] Includes single-donor transfusion products.

[b] Among the 4,984 patients receiving single-donor transfusion products the sources of blood were unspecified regarding 30 including 3 who developed hepatitis.

The widespread acceptance of Titmuss's conclusion that national differences in the incidence of transfusion hepatitis exist and are explained by the use of commercial donors is evidence of strong prior beliefs about the deficiencies of commercialism. According to Titmuss, the reason that the incidence of hepatitis from blood transfusions is lower in England than in the United States is that in England blood is collected from relatively hepatitis free donors, while in the United States some of the blood purchased comes from those members of our society who have extremely high, perhaps the highest, *a priori* probability of having had hepatitis and thus of having contaminated blood.[22]

Some, but far from all, of our purchased blood has been acquired from the derelicts of our society, drug addicts, alcoholics, and prisoners. The difference in the incidence of hepatitis in the blood of paid and unpaid donors is correlated with social status. Transfused blood in England is supplied completely, according to Titmuss, by unpaid altruistic donors. Given this evidence, Titmuss concludes that it is the system of paid donors that is the source of our difficulties and more broadly, the price mechanism which is responsible for many of our social ills.[23] Solow concurs in the view that the use of paid donors is the source of our difficulties. "We can all agree on one point, that the use of paid donors must be responsible for the substantial and growing risk of hepatitis from transfusion."[24] This analysis is not without its apparent impact. In Illinois, paid donor blood has been virtually outlawed as a result of a blood labeling law enacted in 1972, which subjects physicians and hospitals transfusing commercial blood to greater risk of lawsuits and burdens them with additional record keeping. The American Association of Blood Banks is moving towards complete elimination of the use of paid donor blood.[25] "Several states are attempting to pass laws to prohibit *payment for blood.*"[26]

It is widely believed that the *a priori* probability of transmitting serum hepatitis varies by a factor of ten. Despite this expected variation in the quality of blood transfused, price variations that correspond with quality

---

[22] Titmuss implicitly rejects the proposition that a difference in the natural incidence of hepatitis exists. Some evidence exists that supports this view. See Howard F. Taswell, Incidence of HBA_g in Blood Donors: An Overview, in Hepatitis and Blood Transfusion 272.

[23] Glazer accepts this interpretation and suggests that selling blood be outlawed. See Nathan Glazer, Blood, Public Interest No. 24, at 86, 93 (Summer 1971).

[24] Robert M. Solow, *supra* note 7, at 1703.

[25] NHLI Summary Report, at 64.

[26] *Id.* at 2. Outlawing paid donors is supported by the American Red Cross. See Allen Kleiman, Gold Versus the Gift of Blood, 287 New Eng. J. of Med. 51 (1972). In effect the American Red Cross would like to create a new class of victimless crimes.

variations have not been observed in the retail blood market. Moreover, the lowest quality blood seems to travel the greatest distance. Hospital patients are more likely to be offered choices in room accommodations than in the quality of blood transfused.[27] For hospitals dependent upon the single largest supplier of blood, the American National Red Cross, the quality provided has been highly variable. The Red Cross, despite its support of noncommercialism in blood acquisition, has, according to an HEW sponsored study, supplied blood acquired from paid donors.[28] Typically, patients do not have access to information relevant for evaluating the quality of blood to be transfused. Although there exists evidence of significant differences between hospitals with respect to the incidence of hepatitis (hospitals are a proxy for quality), there also exists evidence of great quality differences within particular hospitals and, in the case of multi-unit transfusions, in the quality of the blood transfused to a given patient.[29]

B. The Economics of Blood Supply

Paid blood need not per se be impaired blood. Whether in fact it is impaired depends, as E. R. Jennings has pointed out, not upon whether it was paid for, but from whose veins it comes.[30] There is no reason why paid donors could not come from the same social class that the voluntary donors come from. If so, the two classes of blood would be indistinguishable. Unpaid blood is not, of course, free blood in an economic sense. Advertising, providing a suitable atmosphere for donors, waiting arrangements, opportunity costs of donors' time, etc., are not free.[31]

It is important to recognize that not only in principle is it correct that commercial blood need not be low quality blood, it is true in fact. The world famed Mayo Clinic has a low incidence of transfusion hepatitis and purchases a substantial fraction of the blood its physicians transfuse from suppliers whose sources are the population of small towns in Minnesota.[32] Nor is this an isolated example:

[27] Often there is no explicit charge for blood. More frequently, there is an explicit charge only for blood not replaced by donors provided by the transfused patient.

[28] See NHLI Summary Report, at 134.

[29] See George F. Grady, Ann J. E. Bennett, et al., supra note 21, tabs. 8 & 9, at 697 & 698.

[30] E. R. Jennings, supra note 8, at 8.

[31] Advertising for unpaid donors of blood, which often appear in the editorial pages of the nation's most distinguished newspapers, has a pronounced seasonal pattern that reflects the seasonal pattern in noncommercial giving. There appears to be two seasonal lows in gifts of blood, one around mid-year and the other paradoxically during the Christmas season.

[32] The low incidence in transfusion hepatitis is confirmed by George F. Grady, Ann J. E. Bennett, et al., supra note 21, tab. 9, at 698.

Due to the University's location in a comparatively small town of about 50,000 inhabitants, we are greatly dependent on outside sources of blood and blood components. Because of the increasing awareness of the transmission of hepatitis by transfusion of "commercial" blood, blood banks throughout the country have been rapidly decreasing the use of blood from paid donors in an effort to avoid this problem. Similar trends have been evident at the University of Iowa even though the commercial sources of blood used seemed remarkably free of hepatitis risk. The largest amount of commercial blood was purchased in 1967 when almost 7,600 pints of blood were obtained from such sources. After that time this source of supply has been reduced gradually until April, 1972, when University Hospitals stopped using any commercial blood.[33]

This switch from paid donor to volunteer blood, it is significant to note, occurred despite what are regarded as good results with paid donor blood.[34]

In principle one cannot say whether unpaid blood is cheaper (when blood is explicitly purchased, prices seem to range from five dollars to thirty dollars a unit), as measured by the economic value of the resources used in blood acquisition, or more expensive than paid blood.[35] The evidence presented by Titmuss and confirmed by other investigators indicates that the derelicts of society produce low quality blood and probably should not be paid as much for their blood as their middle class cousins receive. Unless one is prepared to argue that the supply of good quality blood is completely insensitive to price, the evidence presented earlier suggests that a shift away from sources of low quality to sources of high quality blood would reduce the economic costs of medical procedures involving transfusions. Moreover, this shift would seem to be profitable at prices substantially higher than prices currently paid. Low quality blood is, at the margin, more expensive than high quality blood. It is difficult to rationalize the use of low quality blood for anyone who has not had hepatitis. Moreover, if blood costs are covered by third party payers, it is virtually impossible to explain its use.[36]

The experience with transfusion hepatitis suggests that the way to mini-

[33] John A. Koepke (Medical Director, Transfusion Service, University of Iowa Hospitals and Clinics, Iowa City, Iowa), The Variables Affecting Blood Costs in a Large Multi-Source Transfusion Service, in Tri-State Blood Bank Ass'n, First National Symposium on Blood Banking Costs 23, 24 (May, 1973).

[34] Others also report good results with commercial blood. See William V. Miller, Paid Blood Donors, 286 New. Eng. J. Med. 895 (1972). The prestigious Massachusetts General Hospital also uses commercial blood. See Morton Grove-Rasmussen, Gold Versus the Gift of Blood: Fact versus Fiction, 287 New Eng. J. Med. 360 (1972).

[35] The NHLI's study, vol. 1, supra note 4, at 131, reports that the after-tax profit margin of a proprietary blood bank studied was less than that of some of the not-for-profit blood banks.

[36] Feldstein argues that medical insurance has induced undesirable increases in the quality of services provided by the medical establishment, particularly hospitals. The evidence on blood fails to sustain this view. See Martin S. Feldstein, The Medical Economy, in Scientific Am., Sept., 1973, at 151, 154.

mize its incidence is to (1) solicit donors from the socio-economic classes that have a low *a priori* probability of having hepatitis, (2) test for the presence of the hepatitis associated antigen, (3) have a donor pool that is as small as possible consistent with not endangering the health of donors and obtaining the output of blood desired, (4) utilize the information obtained when a transfused patient incurs hepatitis to eliminate tainted blood suppliers from the donor pool.[37]

The foregoing suggest screening would-be donors by socio-economic class and developing sources of blood from regions of the country with a low natural incidence of hepatitis.[38] And within any particular region, there exists evidence that inhabitants of slums have a higher rate than in suburbs. Perhaps the clearest evidence of the differential incidence of hepatitis exists for drug addicts vis-à-vis the nonaddict population: ". . . there are abundant data indicating that narcotic addiction is the principal cause of the high HBA_g-positive rate among people who sell their blood."[39] The foregoing suggests that much of the difference between commercial and noncommercial blood in transmitting serum hepatitis is accounted for by the presence of addicts in the population of commercial donors.

There apparently exists little or no utilization of the knowledge about the incidence of hepatitis in a donor pool from transfused patients who subsequently contract serum hepatitis.[40] Utilization of this knowledge presents some problems—many, if not most, transfusions utilize the blood of more than one donor. Hence new entrants in donor pools should have their blood used in relatively small transfusions or with the blood of other donors for whom there exists, based on past history, a great deal of evidence that they supply hepatitis-free blood. The blood of new entrants in a pool probably ought to be used in transfusions involving children where the risks and hence the costs of hepatitis are low.[41] This, of course, suggests that the value of a donor's

[37] The normal or accepted shelf life of whole blood is twenty-one days. However, for open-heart surgery, there is a premium for fresh blood, because its oxygen-carrying capacity decays with time. Hence the economic value of blood declines monotonically with age. See NHLI's Summary Report, at 138.

[38] See R. Y. Dodd, *et al.*, American National Red Cross Experience with HBA_g Testing, in Hepatitis and Blood Transfusion, 175, 177 reports, based on the presence of HBA_g antigen, a variation of from .2 per 1000 in Waterloo, Iowa, to 3.44 per 1000 in Puerto Rico. For cities an incidence of .29 per 1000 in St. Paul, Minnesota and 3.10 per 1000 in Savannah, Georgia are reported.

[39] Thomas C. Chalmers, Carrier Blood Donors, in Hepatitis and Blood Transfusion 281.

[40] *Id.* at 285-86.

[41] George F. Grady, Ann J. E. Bennett, *et al.*, *supra* note 21; and J. Garrott Allen & Wynn A. Sayman, *supra* note 8, suggest that the lethality of transfusion hepatitis rises with age.

blood, whether or not it is explicitly recognized through a pricing mechanism, rises as the number of hepatitis-free transfusions he supplies increases.

C. Present Arrangements for Supplying Blood

1. *Introduction*

There exist great regional variations in the extent to which commercial blood, that is, blood bought and paid for with dollars, is utilized. Seattle, as previously noted, is on a completely voluntary system.[42] Until relatively recently and for the country as a whole, about one-third of all whole blood transfused was obtained from commercial donors.[43] This is the blood that is generally regarded as the source of much if not most of the serum hepatitis contracted and is being phased out as a source of whole blood for transfusions.

The opposition to commercialism in blood supply is an opposition to the facade of commercialism, not to its substance.[44] Blood assurance programs— which are being expanded—constitute an arrangement by which blood today is bartered for the assurance of blood in the future.[45] A donor, by supplying blood periodically, guarantees blood supplies for himself and his family in the future should they be desired for medical purposes. Similarly patients receiving transfusions are charged "replacement" fees for the blood they receive which are forgiven if they can get enough friends and relatives to replace the blood received. (The rate of transformation of blood so "donated" to blood received often exceeds one-to-one.) Indeed, there are efforts afoot to get insurance companies, particularly Blue Cross, not to cover the cost of blood transfusions in order to induce the friends and relatives of a patient receiving transfusions to "donate" blood.[46] Less than ten per cent of all blood used in the United States is, in Titmuss's language, altruistically given.[47]

[42] Constance Holden, Blood Banking: Money is at the Root of the System's Evils, 175 Science 1344, 1347 (1972).

[43] Richard M. Titmuss, *supra* note 1, at 94.

[44] There seems to be a lack of symmetry in the opposition to commercialism in the procurement of whole blood as distinguished from blood derivative products such as plasma and fibrinogen which also transmit transfusion hepatitis. Typically blood derivative products or components are supplied by commercial drug companies who use the services of paid donors in order to obtain the necessary raw materials. The drive is to eliminate the commercial donor as a source of whole blood but not plasma and fibrinogen. See An Evaluation of the Utilization of Human Blood Resources in the United States 22 (Nat'l Academy of Sciences, Nat'l Res. Council, 1970).

[45] One source estimates that replacement donors at an inner city hospital serving a low-income population have an incidence of HBA_g, the hepatitis-associated antigen whose presence in blood is believed to be highly correlated with the capability of transmitting long incubation hepatitis, about two and a half times greater than the same type of donor at a hospital serving a higher income group. See Howard F. Taswell, *supra* note 22.

[46] See Ron Hasterok, The Insurance Viewpoint on Blood Services, and Arlene E. Kane,

Clearly the opposition is not to commercialism per se in the acquisition of blood for transfusions, but only a certain aspect of commercialism—the payment for blood intermediated by money.[48] The opposition to commercialism intermediated by monetary transactions can be rationalized if one accepts the premise that this type of transaction is a proxy for the acquisition of tainted blood and a finer discrimination against tainted blood would cost more than its benefits. (It is also important that there be no easy transference from one category of commercialism to another.)

It is difficult to accept this explanation because there seems to be no reason why drug addicts, derelicts, prisoners and others with a high *a priori* probability of having hepatitis cannot be screened out directly. Furthermore, the evidence provided by the Mayo Clinic and the Iowa City Blood Bank shows that they can be screened out easily.[49] What then is the explanation for the almost uniform opposition to the acquisition of blood by direct payment?

It is the thesis of this paper that avoiding liability for transfusion hepatitis by the medical establishment explains the opposition to "commercialism" in acquiring blood to be transfused. Eliminating commercialism in blood acquisition is an important plank in the program of the medical establishment for eliminating strict liability in tort for blood.

The recent history of litigation and legislation in Illinois constitutes a

---

The 'Non-Replacement Fee' as a Source of Income, in Tri-State Blood Bank Ass'n, *supra* note 33, at 64 and 103. Many Blue Cross-Blue Shield contracts do not cover the cost of blood. J. Garrott Allen, Commercial Blood in Our National Blood Program, 102 Archives of Surgery 122, 124 (1971) apparently opposes the insurance of blood costs on the grounds that the absence of insurance would encourage "voluntarism" in the supply of blood.

The Southern California Kaiser pre-paid plans, and this is probably true of Kaiser plans in other areas, are not pre-paid with respect to blood. If transfused blood is not replaced, then a replacement fee of twenty-five dollars is charged. Similarly, Medicare does not cover the first three units of a transfusion creating incentives to engage in barter.

Even in Seattle where replacement fees are not levied, the King County Blood Bank makes a great effort to get relatives of patients receiving transfusions to donate blood. The cost of collection and solicitation of blood is buried in a processing charge that includes the cost of cross matching and testing for the presence of the hepatitis associated antigen. Hence, although there is no formal charge for blood, there is a de facto blood charge.

[47] See Marc A. Franklin, Tort Liability for Hepatitis, *supra* note 8, at 441, n.13.

[48] It should be made clear that Titmuss opposed all forms of commercialism in the procurement of blood and the foregoing is meant to describe the views of the American medical establishment which has adopted the facade but not the substance of Titmuss's position.

[49] This does not imply that these organizations are consciously screening. It could simply be attributable to their location in a relatively hepatitis-free area and acquiring blood locally. But it does indicate that by confining blood donors to those in certain socio-economic classes or areas, it is possible to make large reductions in the probability of giving hepatitis producing blood to patients.

piece of evidence in support of the foregoing thesis. In *Cunningham v. Mac-Neal Memorial Hospital*, the State Supreme Court upheld a decision of a lower court that strict liability in tort held in the case of a patient, Francis Cunningham, who had contracted serum hepatitis as a result of a transfusion received at MacNeal Memorial which left the patient with permanent disabilities.[50]

As a result of this decision, organized medicine in Illinois, in particular the hospitals, medical societies and blood suppliers, lobbied for and won from the State Legislature exemption from strict liability in tort for blood.[51] Part of the legislative package won by organized medicine is a blood labeling law. This law burdens physicians transfusing commercial blood. (Explanations of why commercial blood was used must be provided in medical records.) As a result of the blood labeling law, commercial blood is now only rarely used in Illinois, and its use occurs only when noncommercial blood is unavailable. Most states have laws exempting the medical establishment from strict liability for transfusion hepatitis and those that do not are contemplating such laws.[52] The State of Washington provides for strict liability for transfused blood only if the donor is compensated, that is, paid with money, and Idaho provides for liability if the donor is compensated or if the blood bank is a for-profit organization.[53]

This legislation, whose enactment runs counter to the trend towards greater product liability declares that the commercial standards of supplier responsibility typically observed in the product market are inoperative for blood. Although caveat emptor is dying in product markets, particularly those served by profit seeking organizations, it is experiencing a renaissance in the blood market.[54] Some of the reasons advanced for this legislation, which is

[50] Cunningham v. MacNeal Memorial Hospital, 47 Ill. 2d 443, 226 N.E.2d 897 (1970).

[51] The legislation produced is: Ill. Rev. Stat. ch. 111½, §§ 620-1 *et seq.* Florida seems to have followed a similar pattern. In March, 1967, the Florida State Supreme Court ruled that strict liability in tort held for blood in a case similar to the Cunningham case. See Richard M. Titmuss, *supra* note 1, at 162, n.2. Subsequently, legislative relief from the ruling of the court was obtained. See NHLI, Summary Report at 85-86.

[52] NHLI Summary Report at 86. 120 Modern Hospitals, March, 1973, at 48, reports that 45 states have such laws. They define a transfusion of blood as a service and not a product. This is also the position of the American College of Legal Medicine; see Arthur Colemen & James R. Abernathy, Legal Evolution Strikes Blood Banking and Hospitals, 64 J. Nat'l Med. Ass'n 469, 470 (1972).

[53] NHLI Summary Report at 86, Exhibit XXI. The Washington legislation, enacted in 1971, came about as a result of a suit, Reilly v. King County Blood Bank, 6 Wash. App. 172, 492 P.2d 246 (1971), in which strict liability in tort was declared operative for transfusion hepatitis.

[54] Two articles (David L. Rados, Product Liability: Tougher Ground Rules, Harv. Bus. Rev., July-August, 1969, at 144; and Lawrence A. & Arnold I. Bennigson, Product Liability: Manufacturers Beware!, *id.*, May-June, 1974, at 122) argue that caveat emptor

supported by the Red Cross in addition to the medical establishment, is that strict liability for tort will raise the price of blood.[55] But this should not, of course, determine policy; what matters are the full costs of treatment in cluding the costs associated with serum hepatitis. This position can have merit only if the increased price of blood exceeds the reduction in costs of those (a) unfortunate enough to contract transfusion hepatitis and (b) who avoid contracting hepatitis as a result of strict liability.

An argument advanced in support of exemption is the absence of any way of being sure that any particular unit of blood is hepatitis-free. The Illinois Supreme Court rejected this argument in the Cunningham case. The Court held that the same defense applies to typhoid bacilli in clams sold commercially; there is no way of being sure they are not present. Nevertheless, it shall be argued here, they correctly upheld the applicability of the strict liability doctrine.[56]

As a practical matter, strict liability in tort for blood does not exist in the United States. In the states in which legislatures have not granted exemptions to the medical establishment, they have not been needed; the courts have accepted either the view that hospitals are charities and not business establishments or that it is "inherently" impossible to be absolutely certain of blood quality given the present state of knowledge or that blood transfusion is a service and not a product.[57] Only for prepaid groups, the so-called health

---

has been replaced with caveat venditor in the latest ten to fifteen years. For a similar interpretation of trends in the real estate market, see, Robert Kratovil, Courts Shift Their Stance on Real Estate, The Guarantor (Chicago Title & Trust Co., Winter, 1974).

This trend in product liability has implications for the behavior of casualty insurance premiums over time as well as the measurement and/or interpretation of time series of prices.

[55] See the letter by James B. Hartney, M.D., who was Chairman of the Chicago Medical Society's Blood Bank Committee, in the Chicago Tribune, October 17, 1970, at sec. 1, p. 10, col. 5. Also Marc A. Franklin, Hepatitis, Blood Transfusion and Public Action, *supra* note 8, at 702, n.86.

The American Red Cross maintains two positions that appear to be inconsistent. They support outlawing commercial donors in order to protect transfused patients. Yet they simultaneously oppose product liability for blood.

[56] Cunningham v. MacNeal Memorial Hospital, 47 Ill. 2d 443, 266 N.E.2d 897, 902 (1970). An even stronger position supporting strict liability was taken by the Court in Hoffman v. Misericordia Hospital of Philadelphia, 439 Pa. 501, 267 A.2d 867 (1970).

Marilyn J. Ireland, The Legal Framework of the Market for Blood, in the Economics of Charity, 176 & ff. (Institute of Economic Affairs, 1973) has overlooked the legislation nullifying the judicial decisions that held for strict liability. She therefore concluded that product liability exists in these states and as a consequence, the quality of blood either has been or will be improved. In this same volume, David B. Johnson, recognizes the existence of these legislative enactments. *Id.* at 163.

[57] Marc A. Franklin, Tort Liability for Hepatitis, *supra* note 8, at 474, asserts only 9 states still regulate liability for transfusion hepatitis under common law. The remainder, 41, have enacted statutes to limit such liability to negligence. Franklin's count is greater

maintenance organizations, is there any liability at all. Because of their contractual obligations, they bear some, but far from all, of the costs of transfusion hepatitis of their subscribers.

It is clear that the views of legal scholars who have studied product liability have not been sought by state legislators. Calabresi and Bass declare: ". . . what seems clear is that the last person whom we would want to see bear the costs is the individual patient who is unlucky enough to get the bad blood."[58] They regard the incentive to discover better tests of the purity of blood as the principal allocative effect of their view on where liability should be placed.[59] They do not consider the possibility that liability rules can reduce the social or economic costs of serum hepatitis or the therapeutic choice between whole blood and blood components. In this important sense, they differ from the views espoused here or in Franklin's papers.

2. Implications of Coase's Work for Liability Rules

In the abstract zero transactions cost world that Coase investigates in the first part of his famous paper, it is irrelevant where liability is placed because one can costlessly contract out of any initial legal position.[60] The choice of the initial position does not affect the allocation of resources. If liability for serum hepatitis is placed on the physician, then his fees to patients being transfused will be sufficiently higher to pay for the expected costs of the liabilities being incurred. If liability is placed on the patient, then the physician's fees will be lower and the difference in physician fees in these two instances will pay for the expected costs of the risks of hepatitis that are assumed. Similar analysis is relevant and probably more appropriate for hospitals and blood suppliers. (The defendants in the Illinois, Pennsylvania, Florida and Washington cases were either hospitals, blood suppliers, or both.) It is on a

---

than the count of the NHLI Summary Report, despite the fact that the Summary Report has a later publication date and the trend has been towards greater state intervention. A later count in Modern Hospitals, March 1973, at 49, has the number up to 45.

Hospital Week, published by the American Hospital Association, reports that the California appellate court has affirmed a lower court decision and ruled that the transfusion of blood is a service and not the sale of a product. 9 Hospital Week, Aug. 10, 1973.

[58] Guido Calabresi & Kenneth C. Bass, Right Approach, Wrong Implications: A Critique of McKeon on Products Liability, 38 U. Chi. L. Rev. 74, 86 (1970). Franklin does not cite Calabresi and Bass on this point and seems to have, not surprisingly, reached similar conclusions. He devotes a lot of space in this Stanford Law Review article, supra note 8, to the question: Where in the medical establishment—the hospital, physician, blood bank—should liability be placed? In his Catholic University Law Review article, supra note 8, he views with regret the fact that most courts have been immobilized by statutory controls from imposing liability for hepatitis upon the medical establishment.

[59] Guido Calabresi & Kenneth C. Bass, supra note 58, at 84.

[60] R. H. Coase, The Problem of Social Cost, 3 J. Law & Econ. 1 (1960).

par with buying a car with the choice of a one or a two year warranty with appropriate differences in price. If one buys a car with a one year warranty, then liability for the second year is borne by the owner. By contrast, buying a car with a two year warranty implies the seller bears the liability in the second year.

Where liability in the foregoing world is placed is an accounting detail. It is very hard to believe this full knowledge, transaction-cost free world is a prototype for the blood market. The costs incurred by the medical establishment in escaping from liability for tainted blood—there is no free legislation —suggests that they have a strong stake, presumably financial, in avoiding liability for hepatitis.

In recent years there has been a tremendous shift in liability to the hospital and physician from the patient.[61] This shift, in part a result of the development of *Res Ipsa Loquitur* and the greater availability of expert witnesses for plaintiffs, has been opposed on the grounds that it encourages the practice of defensive medicine. Whatever the merits of this argument in other contexts, it is difficult to apply it to blood procurement. Strict liability in tort for serum hepatitis, a form of product liability, does not involve showing whether or not the medical establishment behaved prudently, according to acceptable standards, etc. If a patient is transfused and subsequently becomes ill with transfusion hepatitis, then liability is established. What sorts of records the hospital and/or the attending physician maintained, who he consulted, what tests he ran, are irrelevant. It is not necessary to demonstrate negligence. Hence it is difficult to visualize any role for defensive medicine in warding off liability for tainted blood. Moreover, it is difficult to see how the cost of conducting business between the patient and the physician or the hospital can increase if liability is shifted from the patient.[62]

Is there an argument from the individual consumer's or patient's point of view for not having liability for medical malpractice imposed upon the medical establishment? Would such an imposition increase the relevant costs of blood for consumers by forcing them to buy a higher quality of blood than they desire? For the small class who already have known immunity to transfusion hepatitis, there exists a case for arguing that such legislation is against their interests. Because of the large amounts of blood used in treating hemophilia, a substantial fraction of all hemophiliacs have contracted serum hepa-

---

[61] Between 1960 and 1970, premiums for physicians increased six-fold; surgeons ten-fold; and hospitals three-fold. See the appendix to U.S. Dep't Health, Ed. & Welfare, Report of the Secretary's Commission on Medical Malpractice 48 (January 16, 1973).

[62] The argument Coase used in explaining the opposition to imposing liability upon railroads for fire damage to crops along the right of way, formidable costs of transacting between the railroad and farmers, seems to be inapplicable here. See R. H. Coase, *supra* note 60, at 31.

titis in the past and are immune to this ailment.[63] Hemophiliacs with immunity to serum hepatitis constitute the only natural market for low quality addict blood. Hence, they would lose unless they could recontract with health care providers to assume the risk of hepatitis and this market was large enough to be catered to by blood suppliers.[64]

3. *Where Should Liability Be Placed?*

Consider a situation in which liability is placed on a patient and he buys and pays for blood with three chances in one thousand of incurring hepatitis per unit purchased. Further assume that he subsequently contracts transfusion hepatitis. It is very difficult *ex post* to determine whether or not he bought three chances in one thousand blood or three chances in one hundred. He has an expensive and virtually insurmountable gap in knowledge to overcome, particularly in a world in which data on the incidence of hepatitis is not easy to come by, in finding out whether or not the product purchased is in fact the product delivered. Hence, civil remedies are virtually precluded unless strict liability exists.

Moreover, it must not be forgotten that not all blood is transfused as a result of elective surgery or other elective procedures. A non-trivial fraction of all blood is transfused to patients that are found in trauma as a result of accidents and are in no position to weigh alternatives in the blood market. Under such circumstances, it is somewhat ludicrous to expect patients to take responsibility for the quality of the blood they receive; whatever virtues caveat emptor may have in other contexts, it is difficult to argue that it should prevail here.

Both the physician and the hospital can more cheaply obtain the knowledge required to determine whether the quality of blood ordered for a patient is in fact received. They are in a better position, as compared with the patient, to obtain the information relevant for evaluating the medical experiences of all patients transfused with blood from a particular supplier. Hence, if liability is placed with either the hospital or the physician, which almost surely will involve some subsequent transference to the blood supplier, those who have the cheapest access to the relevant information will be making the choice and evaluating the performance of blood suppliers. This information will be used in setting fees and hospital charges to the patient who in turn

[63] See Blood Banking—Major Findings by HEW Task Force 5, in U.S. Dep't of Health, Ed. & Welfare, Conference on the National Blood Policy (unpublished reports, 1973).

[64] Presumably physicians or hospitals might also want to contract with blood banks to transfer some of the liability for serum hepatitis. In Illinois, hemophiliacs have won, through the exercise of political muscle, the right to barter blood donated on their behalf, by friends, relatives and others, for hospital costs they incur. For everyone else, blood can only be bartered for blood.

will be in a better position to evaluate alternatives in the medical care market than he would be if he were self-insured.

The case for placing liability directly on the physician rather than on the hospital or the blood supplier rests on the fact that he chooses among alternative modes of treatment. Hence he is in the best position to evaluate whether blood or blood substitutes ought to be used, and in what quantities, and to evaluate the risks to specific patients. Therefore, he can, at a lower cost than anyone else, obtain the information relevant for decisions involving the risks of hepatitis and compare them with other medical risks.

4. Why is Strict Liability Opposed?

If defensive medicine, which raises the costs of medical care without a commensurate increase in the utility of medical care to consumers, is rejected as a rationale for the opposition of the suppliers of medical care to the transference of liability from the patient to the suppliers, how is this opposition to be explained? The imposition of product liability upon the consumer is the result of a coalition between the medical societies, hospitals, and blood banks. The blood legislation won by this coalition is a testimonial to its political power. However the question remains: Why was this legislation sought?

Eliminating caveat emptor from the blood market would require the current suppliers of blood to adapt to a wholly new set of rules for survival. Whenever liability is placed on the supply side of the medical care market, it is bound to be shifted around so that the supplier of blood will have to effectively guarantee the quality of the product supplied. Hence, standards of supplier responsibility which are characteristic of commercial markets, in particular the drug market, will be imposed upon charitable institutions such as the American Red Cross or hospital blood banks.

Currently the comparative advantage of these organizations in the blood market is solicitation, that is, begging for blood and money. The value of this comparative advantage in a market in which suppliers could not evade product liability would decline sharply; indiscriminate solicitation, because the donor pool is so large, yields too much tainted blood. Hence, imposing strict liability upon these volunteer agencies would be on a par with permitting the practice of nudism only in the polar regions; it is doubtful the cult could survive the rigours of this constraint. Since the supply of blood is the principal product line of the American Red Cross and many other groups such as the King County Blood Bank in Seattle, their place in the sun would either be eliminated or sharply reduced. Therefore, it is not difficult to understand why both the hospitals and blood suppliers (and many hospitals are blood suppliers) oppose strict liability.

The opposition of the medical profession to strict liability is more difficult to understand.[65] The American Red Cross and hospital and community blood banks prefer, in common with most economic enterprises, to exclude competitors. However, for the medical profession, blood is a complementary resource like hospitals. Hence, it appears to be in the self-interest of physicians for a highly competitive blood market to exist. Consequently, promoting voluntarism for blood donors, fighting product liability, and working to eliminate commercial donors does not appear to make economic sense.

What then is the explanation of the position of the AMA? Marshall's theory of joint demand implies that the lower the prices of resources complementary to the services of a monopolist, the higher the monopoly returns. Hence for medicine which is characterized by highly restricted entry and monopoly returns, there exists strong economic incentives to promote economic conditions that minimize the costs of blood for every quality level. In a subsidy free world, this would surely be a highly competitive blood market.

It is important to recognize that within the membership of the AMA are physicians associated with both the production and the consumption of blood. As employees of blood banks, physicians are overrepresented among banks using volunteer blood. Per unit of blood produced by blood banks, those using volunteer blood employ relatively physician-intensive procedures. Indeed, standards for the accreditation of blood banks have been set up that require that these organizations be run by physicians if not pathologists.[66] Hence, the job opportunities of these physicians are threatened by commercialism in the supply of blood.

The interests of physicians engaged in the production of blood, in contrast to the interests of the general membership of the AMA, is to drive commercialism out of the blood business. Moreover, the interests of these physicians are concentrated whereas the interests of the general membership in a competitive blood market are diffuse. It is not unusual in political organizations to find that the interests of producers are overrepresented relative to consumers because the transactions costs in making diffuse consumer interests politically effective are greater than they are for concentrated producer interests. In other words, the decision-making structure of the AMA with respect to blood is dominated by producer interests that are employed by blood banks using volunteer blood.

As a result of the political power of the coalition of physicians, hospitals,

---

[65] Organized medicine has expressed its opposition to strict liability for blood in an editorial entitled Blood Money, in 215 J. Am. Med. Ass'n 109-110 (Jan. 1971). Its support for voluntarism appears in Am. Medical Ass'n, Comm. on Transfusion & Transplantation, Guide for Hospital Committee on Transfusion 3 (undated).

[66] See NHLI Study, vol. 1, *supra* note 4, at 373.

and volunteer blood banks, product liability for blood-derivative products, some supplied by large national drug companies, are either in doubt or non-existent. Many blood derivative products, such as plasma and fibrinogen, are supplied by both voluntary agencies such as the Red Cross and commercial drug companies and, like whole blood, have the capability of transmitting transfusion hepatitis. The laws declaring blood transfusions to be a service and not a product also declare or imply that the transfusion of blood derivatives is a service and not a product. (In Illinois, all blood derivative products are exempt by statute even if supplied by an avaricious and highly profitable drug company.) Hence, the usual commercial standards of supplier responsibility for drug products exacted from the drug companies are suspended for blood derivatives. However, even if the normal commercial standards were applied to drug companies for blood derivative products, the exemption for whole blood creates difficult problems in assessing liability because whole blood and blood derivatives are often jointly used to treat patients.

5. Why is Too Low Quality of Blood Now Being Provided?

If the figures on the marginal value of low risk over high risk blood are correct, then there still remains the question: Why have not hospitals developed better sources of blood? After all, both physicians and hospitals are concerned with the welfare of their patients. A large part of the answer to this question must be that the dangers of transfusion hepatitis are relatively new on the medical scene and neither patients nor physicians are as alert to this problem currently as they will be when more experience with this complication of transfusions is accumulated. Hence, one can argue that in the long run, the Coase theorem will hold. Under this interpretation, suppliers of blood should be currently moving in the direction of improving blood quality.

A role of strict liability, given the foregoing interpretation, is to influence the pace at which the medical establishment adjusts to the relatively recently developed knowledge about the relationship of blood sources to the transmission of transfusion hepatitis. Currently whether or not a hospital develops good sources seems to be relatively insensitive to pressures from either patients or physicians. Grady asserts:

. . . in my experience, most hospitals have been successful in improving the quantity and quality of their blood sources only insofar as it was of concern to the local prime figure in the clinical teaching and bedside care hierarchy. For example, if the Chief of Surgery of an outstanding surgical service thinks it is important to have low risk blood, it is usually provided by one means or another. If hepatitis risk is considered a relatively minor problem and has to compete and take its place among thousands of other problems, then improvements are unlikely in spite of technological advances. It is simply a question of leadership.[67]

Because of the absence of advertising competition among hospitals, the fact that some hospitals are alert to the dangers of hepatitis to their patients and obtain low risk blood does not force other hospitals to find sources of blood of equal quality in order to remain economically viable. Hence the claims and litigation arising out of the existence of strict liability are especially important in this particular market as a means of exerting pressure on the prime figures in the medical hierarchy of hospitals to obtain low risk blood. Strict liability would reduce the survival properties of hospitals with a medical hierarchy that was insensitive to or ignorant of the risks of hepatitis for their patients. Consequently, they would move faster towards providing the quality of blood their patients want.

In the absence of strict liability, the pace at which the medical establishment will move towards providing low risk blood for patients will be much slower. Eventually enough information is generated by the experience of relatives and friends, by articles and books, by radio and TV, and by newspapers so that both the public and physicians, both sides of the market, will become informed of the risks and only low risk blood will be used. This is a more expensive way of disseminating the relevant information, hence the movement towards long-run equilibrium will be slower than it would be if strict liability existed.

The desire to avoid product liability explains the inconsistency between the opposition to commercialism in blood procurement on the one hand and the promotion of barter as a means of providing blood on the other. In order to avoid product liability, the patient is induced to provide his own blood via blood assurance programs and the hospital provides transfusion services. For the same reason medical insurors controlled by the medical establishment, such as Blue Cross and Blue Shield, do not provide coverage of blood costs, nor do many pre-paid groups, that is the so-called health maintenance organizations. They all wish to establish that the provision of blood is a service and not a product. The desire to avoid product liability also explains why the medical establishment has not imposed quality standards upon their blood suppliers. Such standards would inevitably be defined in terms of the risks of

---

[67] G. F. Grady, HBA$_g$ in Blood Donors, in Hepatitis and Blood Transfusion 310. It should be pointed out that Grady must be regarded as a relatively knowledgeable observer since he is the senior author of one of the most, if not the most, extensive empirical studies of the relationship between blood sources and transfusion hepatitis using data derived from many hospitals. Hence he ought to be well aware of hospital procurement practices.

hepatitis and therefore would increase the risks that courts and/or legislators would impose similar standards upon the medical establishment.

A test of the explanation offered for the unwillingness of the medical establishment to accept strict liability in tort for blood is provided by the legislation in Idaho and Washington which imposes strict liability if commercial blood is transfused. One would expect if the hypothesis presented is correct, that the frequency with which commercial blood is used in these two states will be significantly lower than it is for the country as a whole. Blood procurement practices in both of these states support this implication.

Whether or not blood is obtained from volunteers, paid donors, or altruistic donors in the Titmuss sense of the term, is irrelevant. Similarly, whether or not paid donors drive altruistic donors out of business is also irrelevant.[68] What is relevant is the quality of blood transfused and the incentive to obtain good blood for this purpose. Imposing strict liability upon the attending physician or the hospital or the blood supplier will accelerate the achievement of this end. By virtue of this liability there will be additional financial incentives, incentives that have been absent, to obtain less dangerous blood for transfusions. The drug addict, but not necessarily the paid donor, will be driven out of the blood business as a result of efforts to keep malpractice insurance costs and premiums down. This conclusion should hold if liability is placed upon physicians, whether or not they contract out some or all of their liability to either hospitals or blood banks.[69]

The additional financial incentives of strict liability will mobilize the resources of the market to find and utilize economical supplies of high quality blood.[70] Probably a thoroughgoing system of professional blood donors will develop, professionals being usually better than amateurs. The analysis presented implies that voluntarism in blood procurement is a *deus ex machina* which makes possible the anomalous rule of liability for blood that currently prevails. Hence imposing strict liability for blood would eliminate voluntarism and explains the hostility towards commercial blood procurement by voluntary agencies.

[68] The theorem that in one market only one price can exist implies that paid and unpaid donors cannot simultaneously coexist unless unpaid donors have utility functions that are rare in nature. In the absence of such utility functions, payment for blood will simply increase the producer's surplus of would-be unpaid donors. This suggests that voluntary donors would be recruited by blood donor services willing to pay. Hence, a natural antipathy towards the organizations that pay for blood by institutions such as the Red Cross is implied by this analysis.

[69] Franklin apparently rejects applying strict liability to physicians for reasons difficult to understand. See Marc A. Franklin, Tort Liability for Hepatitis, *supra* note 8, at 472.

[70] There exists some evidence that suggests non-profit hospitals respond relatively slowly to changes in demand conditions. See Bruce Steinwald & Duncan Neuhauser, The Role of the Proprietary Hospital, 1970 Law & Contemp. Prob. 815, 837.

The fact that the Mayo Clinic pays for blood is suggestive of the direction of the medical establishment would move in a world of strict liability.[71] Moreover, more screening by social class, absence or presence of slum background, and medical history would occur. Implicit prices would become explicit; the price of the blood supplied by a given donor would rise as the number of trouble-free units previously supplied increased. Professional donors would have incentives to stay healthy and blood banks would have incentives to weed unsatisfactory donors out of their pools. Moreover, more thought would go into designing programs for administering transfusions that would make it easy and hence less expensive to detect donors of tainted blood.[72]

CONCLUSIONS

It has been argued that Titmuss is correct in the sense that too low a quality of blood has been provided by the medical establishment to patients.[73]

[71] This is not regarded as commercialism by those who study the relationship between blood sources and hepatitis. The Mayo Clinic or the hospitals servicing the Mayo Clinic buy blood from churches in small towns in Minnesota. These churches, in turn, procure this blood as gifts from their members. Hence gifts of blood are an alternative to gifts of money. By giving blood instead of money, church members escape taxes on their earnings as blood donors. If blood were sold directly by donors instead of indirectly through churches, only the aftertax receipts from the sale of blood would be available for church support. Hence taxes are escaped whose magnitude is a function of the marginal tax brackets of donors. This source of blood is defined to be other volunteer donors in George F. Grady, Ann J. E. Bennett, et al., supra note 21, tab. 8, at 697. One can search in vain in this article for the definition of other volunteer donors only.

At times one has the feeling that commercialism is defined as that method of procuring blood that has the highest incidence of transfusion hepatitis. For example, group three in George F. Grady, Ann J. E. Bennett, et al., supra note 21, tab. 8, at 697, is referred to as paid non-commercial donor in Posttransfusion Hepatitis, supra note 15, at 8. This category is ignored by Howard F. Taswell, supra note 22, at 272, when he compares the risks of hepatitis from volunteer and commercial blood. He averages the incidence of hepatitis for the two classes of volunteer donors and compares the number obtained with the risks associated with the blood described in group four. His comparison is more inept than misleading since he fails to adjust for differences in the average size of transfusion.

Commercial blood is defined by the Illinois law as blood obtained from a donor in exchange for money. If blood is not procured from a donor through monetary incentives, it can be subsequently resold an indefinite number of times and still remain non-commercial blood.

[72] The problem of supplying blood is in many ways symmetrical with the problem of supplying semen for artificially inseminating human females. The suppliers of semen are solicited and paid by the medical establishment and effort is expended in discovering males who will provide a high quality set of genes. The usual source is medical students. In the past, they were an important source of blood for transfusions.

[73] The evidence on blood quality is not the only empirical support for Titmuss's view that our blood procurement program works badly. Section III, Blood Banking, in U.S. Dep't Health, Ed., & Welfare supra note 63, at 5, reports that some plasma pools come

Titmuss has interpreted this finding as a consequence of too much commercialism; in our view it is a consequence of too little commercialism. The acquisition of an exemption from product liability for blood by the medical establishment delays the development of low risk sources of blood by emasculating short-run financial incentives to undertake such development.

It is doubtful that many of the institutions involved in blood procurement today, such as the American Red Cross, would be viable in a world in which the usual commercial standards of supplier responsibility existed. Similarly the management of blood procurement by hospitals would become more difficult and hence it is likely that some managers would not be viable in this more difficult world. Hence, there exists powerful special interest groups, apart from physicians, whose economic interests are served by opposing strict liability.

Because of the absence of strict liability, it is possible to observe patients in major hospital centers, all obviously viable producers of open heart surgery, incurring vastly different frequencies of transfusion hepatitis. For example, the two largest producers of open heart surgery in Grady's study, and it is not unlikely that they are the two largest producers in the world, differ by a factor of eight in the incidence of symptomatic hepatitis.[74]

The recommendation for changes in liability rules essentially argues that the standards of product liability taken for granted in the commercial world should be applied to transfused blood. The present liability rule is highly anomalous, exists because of the pressures upon state legislatures by organized medicine and is, in our view, anti-consumer legislation. It is hard to defend caveat emptor for blood but not for cars, soup, and the hundreds of products found in the market place. If state legislatures had not intervened, that is, if they had done nothing, strict liability in tort for blood and blood derivatives would exist in many if not most of the states in the United States. "The

---

from as many as a thousand donors. This implies that the pool is almost certain to be contaminated even if the probability of any one donor's blood being contaminated is on the order of one or two chances in a thousand. Clearly the procedure to follow if one wished to raise the probability of contaminating a pool is to increase its size. It is difficult to believe that government intervention to eliminate the use of pooled plasma would either be necessary or occur in a world in which strict liability for hepatitis existed.

This source also estimates that 25% of all whole blood collected for transfusion is never transfused and most of these non-transfused units are wasted through outdating. This view may also be found in An Evaluation of the Utilization of Human Blood Resources, *supra* note 44, at 21. However, this source, *id.* at 37, suggests that this waste is inherent in voluntarism whereas Titmuss argues that it is produced by commercialism.

[74] George F. Grady, Ann J. E. Bennett, *et al.*, *supra* note 21, tab. 6, at 696 reports a difference of a factor of six. However, the average size of transfusions in the poorer center, Cleveland Clinic, is seven units against over nine in the better one, Mayo Clinic. See *id.* tab. 9, at 698. Of the patients transfused at the poorer center, 3.4% exhibited symptomatic hepatitis. In one of the poorest centers, the rate was 8.1%. *Id.* tab. 6, at 696.

kind of situation which economists (and others) are prone to consider as requiring corrective Government action is, in fact, often the result of Governmental action."[75] The desire to maintain a highly anomalous product liability rule for blood explains why commercial blood is relatively absent in Washington and Idaho. It also explains the opposition to paid donors and the promotion of barter among the potential patient population as a means of acquiring blood for transfusions. Moreover, it explains the lower standards for blood derivative products supplied by drug companies.

It is important to recognize that the long-run supply function of information to patients about the risks of hepatitis from transfusions, or the potential benefits and risks of any other medical procedure is flatter than the short-run supply function. Eventually enough information is generated by the experience of relatives and friends, by articles and books, by radio and TV, and by newspapers so that the public can make relatively accurate evaluations cheaply. However, the transfusion of whole blood is a relatively new medical development growing out of our experience during World War II and the discovery of transfusion hepatitis came relatively recently. Hence if transfusion hepatitis were an old established ailment, the case for strict liability would be weaker but not nonexistent.

Currently the favored method of assuring the provision of low risk blood for transfusions is to regulate donors—more specifically, to outlaw "commercial donors."[76] Hence product liability, a form of direct control over the output of blood suppliers that is enforced by the users of blood, is an alternative to indirect control over inputs of blood suppliers enforced by government regulation. The history of legislation regulating medical care delivery suggests that such regulation of inputs is more likely to represent the interests of the medical establishment than the transfused patient.

[75] R. H. Coase, *supra* note 60, at 28. (Brackets added.)

[76] Volunteer donors are alleged to be better than paid donors because paid donors have an incentive to conceal facts about their health that would make them unacceptable donors. The proponents of this view have not recognized that the same argument is relevant for replacement donors or candidates for membership in blood assurance programs. Indeed, hospitals in areas serving a large number of ghetto dwelling patients who require blood as a result of trauma will probably have low quality blood provided by their replacement donors.

LIST OF PARTICIPANTS

Adams, John G., *Pharmaceutical Manufacturers Association, Washington, D.C.*
Alter, Harvey J., M.D., *National Institutes of Health, Bethesda, Maryland*
Ammerati, Carmine, *Technicon Corporation, Tarrytown, New York*
Ashworth, John, *Cutter Laboratories, Inc., Berkeley, California*
Baiardo, Don, *General Accounting Office, Washington, D.C.*
Bellman, Betty, *JRB Associates, McLean, Virginia*
Broderick, Kathleen, *American National Red Cross, Washington, D.C.*
Burns, Kathleen A., *Towson, Maryland*
Byrne, Robert J., *National Institutes of Health, Bethesda, Maryland*
Caplan, Sorrell, *Communique, Washington, D.C.*
Cardozo, Michael H., *Washington, D.C.*
Carol, Arthur, *Washington, D.C.*
Carr, Edward O., *Central Florida Blood Bank, Orlando, Florida*
Christman, James N., *Hunton & Williams, Richmond, Virginia*
Coe, Norman, *Washington Regional Red Cross Blood Center, Washington, D.C.*
Crispen, James F., M.D., *Harrisburg Polyclinic Hospital, Harrisburg, Pennsylvania*
Dalison, R. Ben, M.D., *University of Maryland Hospital, Baltimore, Maryland*
DeSilva, Joel, *Nicholls State University, Thibodaux, Louisiana*
Dodd, Roger Y., *American National Red Cross, Bethesda, Maryland*
Dolan, William D., M.D., *Arlington, Virginia*
Dougherty, Don T., *Spokane & Inland Empire Blood Bank, Spokane, Washington*
Drees, Thomas C., *Abbott Laboratories, South Pasadena, California*
Dunbar, John, *National Institutes of Health, Bethesda, Maryland*
Ebert, Virginia, *Merck & Co., Inc., West Point, Pennsylvania*
Eisenman, David, *Champaign, Illinois*
Ennis, David, *Blood Bank of Delaware, Inc., Newark, Delaware*
Fitch, David J., *National Center for Health Services Research, DHEW, Rockville, Maryland*
Flowers, Dorothy, *Blue Cross and Blue Shield of Greater New York, New York, New York*
Freilich, William, *Merck & Co., Inc., Rahway, New Jersey*
Friedman, Leonard I., *American National Red Cross, Bethesda, Maryland*
Friest, Philip L., *Blood Donors, Inc., Duluth, Minnesota*
Fry, Robert, *Stewart Blood Center, Inc., Tyler, Texas*
Gary, John H., *Interstate Blood Bank, Inc., Memphis, Tennessee*
Gill, James J., *Harvard University Health Services, Cambridge, Massachusetts*
Goldenberg, Mel, *Hoffmann-La Roche Inc., Cranbury, New Jersey*

Goodwin, Norman, *American National Red Cross, Washington, D.C.*

Gray, Alan I., *Merck Sharp & Dohme, West Point, Pennsylvania*

Greenberg, Warren, *Federal Trade Commission, Washington, D.C.*

Greene, Doris Danzig, *Health Policy Center, Georgetown University*

Grossmueller, Werner, *Ortho Diagnostics Inc., Raritan, New Jersey*

Grupenhoff, John T., *American Society of Hematology, Washington, D.C.*

Gunter, Lt. Col. James J., *USAF, Washington, D.C.*

Heffernan, Henry, *School of Medicine, Georgetown University, Washington, D.C.*

Hemphill, Bernice M., *Irwin Memorial Blood Bank, San Francisco, California*

Jahns, Marsha, *American Hospital Association, Washington, D.C.*

James, Lois J., *American Association of Blood Banks, Washington, D.C.*

Johnson, Robert C., *Armour Pharmaceutical Company, Kankakee, Illinois*

Kammerer, Robert C., *North Jersey Blood Center, East Orange, New Jersey*

Kadar, Geza, Jr., *Blue Cross Association, Washington, D.C.*

Karlson, Robert E., *Ortho Diagnostics Inc., Raritan, New Jersey*

Kear, Norman R., *American National Red Cross Blood Program, Washington, D.C.*

Kennedy, Greg, *Pfizer Diagnostics Division, Groton, Connecticut*

King, George, *Overlook Park, Kansas*

Kyler, William S., *Council of Community Blood Centers, Scottsdale, Arizona*

LaBrec, Eugene, *Electronucleonics Laboratories, Inc., Bethesda, Maryland*

Larson, Paul, *Ortho Diagnostics Inc., Raritan, New Jersey*

Legarven, Paul, *Veterans Administration, Washington, D.C.*

Leonardi, Linda, *Chicago, Illinois*

Lichtiger, Benjamin, M.D., *Anderson Hospital, Texas Medical Center, Houston, Texas*

London, Thomas, *Institute for Cancer Research, National Institutes of Health, Bethesda, Maryland*

Long, Steve, *Franklin and Marshall College, Lancaster, Pennsylvania*

Loosebrock, T.A., *Miller Memorial Blood Center, Bethlehem, Pennsylvania*

Luettgen, Jane, *Milwaukee Blood Center, Milwaukee, Wisconsin*

Martin, Don, *University of Miami School of Law, Coral Gables, Florida*

Massie, Robert, *Princeton University, Princeton, New Jersey*

Masson, Allison, *Federal Trade Commission, Washington, D.C.*

Mathis, Meyer, *American Red Cross, Washington, D.C.*

McCall, Mike, *Travenol Laboratories, Inc., Deerfield, Illinois*

McGarry, Edward C., *Community Blood Bank of Broward County, Fort Lauderdale, Florida*

McIlrath, Sharon, *Blue Cross Association, Washington, D.C.*

Mitchell, William L., *Washington, D.C.*

Miller, Ted R., *American Blood Commission, Arlington, Virginia*

Morse, Edward, M.D., *School of Medicine, University of Connecticut, Farmington, Connecticut*

Mullen, Sanford A., M.D., *Jacksonville Blood Bank, Jacksonville, Florida*

Myhre, Byron A., M.D., *Harbor General Hospital, Torrance, California*

Ni, Louisa, *American National Red Cross, Washington, D.C.*

Payne, Conrad, *American National Red Cross, Washington, D.C.*

Peake, Col. Ben F., *American Association of Blood Banks, Washington, D.C.*

Pearlman, Daniel, *U.S. Department of Justice, Washington, D.C.*

Petit, Caroline, *American Blood Commission, Arlington, Virginia*

Pindus, Nancy M., *American Blood Commission, Arlington, Virginia*

Pisarkiewicz, John, *Federal Trade Commission, Washington, D.C.*

Popkin, Mary, *American Red Cross, Washington, D.C.*

Prete, Douglas, *Richmond Metropolitan Blood Service, Richmond, Virginia*

Rados, David L., *Graduate School of Business, Columbia University, New York, New York*

Raymer, Dorothy, *Chek-Lab, Inc., Aurora, Illinois*

Reilly, Robert W., *Annapolis, Maryland*

Rene, Anthony A., *National Institutes of Health, Bethesda, Maryland*

Reynolds, Doug, *Merck & Co., Inc., Rahway, New Jersey*

Richards, Alan K., *Blue Cross & Blue Shield*

Rodell, Michael, *Hyland Division of Travenol Laboratories, Inc., Costa Mesa, California*

Roll, Fred, *Philadelphia, Pennsylvania*

Romansky, Michael, *Washington, D.C.*

Roser, H.C., Jr., *Exxon Corporation, New York, New York*

Russell, James E., *JRB Associates, McLean, Virginia*

St. Clair, Dennis L., *Boehringer Associates, Wynnewood, Pennsylvania*

Sassetti, Richard J., *Chicago, Illinois*

Sauve, Martha, *American Red Cross, Washington, D.C.*

Savitt, Harry L., *Social Security Administration, Baltimore, Maryland*

Schwartz, Elinor, *Physicians Radio Network, Washington, D.C.*

Schwartz, Harry, *New York Times, New York, New York*

Shinagawa, Emiko, *Irwin Memorial Blood Bank, San Francisco, California*

Simon, Ernest R., M.D., *Food and Drug Administration, Bethesda, Maryland*

Solomon, Joel, M.D., *Food and Drug Administration, Bethesda, Maryland*

Spell, Eva, *Food and Drug Administration, Bethesda, Maryland*

Staub, Donna, *Jacksonville Blood Bank, Jacksonville, Florida*

Stephens, Randall, *American National Red Cross, Washington, D.C.*

Stokes, Goodrich H., *American Hospital Association, Washington, D.C.*

Teague, Bill T., *Gulf Coast Regional Blood Center, Houston, Texas*

Thornton, John L., *Richmond Metropolitan Blood Service, Richmond, Virginia*

Tierney, John T., *State of Rhode Island Health Department, Providence, Rhode Island*

Torrison, Lewis, *American National Red Cross, Washington, D.C.*

Updegraff, Gail, *Food and Drug Administration, Rockville, Maryland*

Vaithianathan, Thiru, M.D., *Chicago, Illinois*

Vogt, Leslie H., *Richmond Metropolitan Blood Service, Richmond, Virginia*

Walsh, Bernadette, *American National Red Cross, Washington, D.C.*

Walter, Carl W., M.D., *Boston, Massachusetts*

Weltman, Robert, *American Medical Association, Washington, D.C.*

Wendlandt, Gay, M.D., *Anderson Hospital and Tumor Institute, Houston, Texas*

West, William G., *Central Blood Bank of Pittsburgh, Pittsburgh, Pennsylvania*

Wickerhauser, Milan, *American National Red Cross, Bethesda, Maryland*

Wilkins, Marilynn G., *DHEW, Rockville, Maryland*

Willett, David E., *San Francisco, California*

Wozmak, Mark, *Central Kentucky Blood Center, Lexington, Kentucky*

Zuelzer, Wolf W., *National Heart and Lung Institute, National Institutes of Health, Bethesda, Maryland*